All-Natural Ways
to Health & Beauty

Kiss Your Doctor Goodbye

ELKE   F.   LEWIS

BALBOA.
PRESS

A DIVISION OF HAY HOUSE

Balboa Press books may be ordered through booksellers or by contacting:

Balboa Press
A Division of Hay House
1663 Liberty Drive
Bloomington, IN 47403
www.balboapress.com
1 (877) 407-4847

Because of the dynamic nature of the Internet, any web addresses or links contained in this book may have changed since publication and may no longer be valid. The views expressed in this work are solely those of the author and do not necessarily reflect the views of the publisher, and the publisher hereby disclaims any responsibility for them.

The author of this book does not dispense medical advice or prescribe the use of any technique as a form of treatment for physical, emotional, or medical problems without the advice of a physician, either directly or indirectly. The intent of the author is only to offer information of a general nature to help you in your quest for emotional and spiritual well-being. In the event you use any of the information in this book for yourself, which is your constitutional right, the author and the publisher assume no responsibility for your actions.

Any people depicted in stock imagery provided by Getty Images are models, and such images are being used for illustrative purposes only. Certain stock imagery © Getty Images.

Scripture taken from the New King James Version. Copyright 1979, 1980, 1982 by Thomas Nelson, inc. Used by permission. All rights reserved.

This book is a work of non-fiction. Unless otherwise noted, the author and the publisher make no explicit guarantees as to the accuracy of the information contained in this book and in some cases, names of people and places have been altered to protect their privacy.

Print information available on the last page.

ISBN: 978-1-5043-9921-0 (sc)
ISBN: 978-1-5043-9923-4 (hc)
ISBN: 978-1-5043-9922-7 (e)

Library of Congress Control Number: 2018902521

Balboa Press rev. date: 02/22/2019

Contents

I dedicate this book with all my love to my husband
Steven Calvin Lewis.

To my beloved puppy angel Chico, who was my joyful companion
for only 8 months,
To Chico's cousin Shanti, who brings me joy every day,
To Carlos, my inspiration and love of my life,

and to all courageous Souls who wish to live a long and healthy
life on earth with the purpose to serve humanity.

Disclaimer

This book is not medical advice. It has been written after the author's many years of professional and personal experience in the field of Nutrition and Natural Self-Healing. Most suggestions are time-proven or of folkloric origin. However, all are anecdotes and the information is for educational purposes only and not intended to prevent, treat, cure or diagnose any disease. Statements or opinions have not been evaluated by the FDA. Each person is unique, and if you have concerns about your health or want to make changes in your diet, your lifestyle, use a new supplement, vitamins or herbs, you should always consult with a physician or other healthcare professional first. Neither the author nor the publishers are responsible for any use of the information presented.

Foreword

Diets have been around ever since mankind existed. In the times of Adam and Eve people did not refer to them as special diets. They ate what was available to them in the Garden of Eden and were content with it. Everything in those times was good and pure, including the air they breathed. There were no cars in Paradise, no TV, no newspaper, no smog, no money, no credit cards, and not much to worry about.

Today, we live in a different environment. It has become almost an art to choose the most appropriate food for our wellbeing in a world where so much is offered. We do not live a pristine environment anymore, and yet the desire for health and happiness is greater than ever. We also tend to think that more is better. We want more food, a bigger house, a faster car, want to go to the most entertaining parties, choose expensive schools for our kids, wear the latest fashion, and go to exotic places on vacation, all for the lowest possible price. After chasing those dreams, and achieving some of them, we might still realize a certain emptiness inside. Everything is good, but on their own these things cannot fulfill us.

It is nice to have "things," but what we truly desire is good health, love, peace, freedom, and above all, more joy in our lives. We want to feel good and look good. Having more money, better health, a good education and beautiful objects can be valuable, but they are not our final goals. However, they may be stepping stones to achieve what is of true value. There are always difficulties on our path, and in a way it is exactly those difficulties that help us learn and grow. When we are sick, we want health. When we experience lack, we want abundance. Limitations awaken our desire. Whatever we want to do, be or have, most of it can be achieved as soon as we take responsibility and start taking action. It is our thoughts, words, and actions that determine what happens in our life. Pleasant experiences could be feedback that we are on the right path, whereas each obstacle, each downfall, each pain is a nudge by the Universe letting us know that it is time to change course. It could also mean: Don't give up! Things are going to change soon. One way or the other, everything is a learning experience helping us to grow stronger and eventually have a better life.

Our health is no exception. Although we can be happy in any situation, good health and beauty can be valuable assets for more joy and advancements. Gaining a better understanding of how our body works, and how it continually talks to us either through pain, wellbeing, or a variety of symptoms, it always guides us to get to the best possible condition. We can learn to slow down the aging process and remain youthful at any age. We have to know what to eat and what to stay away from, and as a general rule we need to keep things simple.

This book is meant to give us guidelines. It covers some of my own experiences. Some guidelines are from ancient scriptures or from other teachers in the health field. Much of it I have learnt from my clients, working over forty years in the field of nutrition and natural health. Sometimes we learn the most from people who at one time were given up on by the medical profession and then found a way to become living examples of health, strength, and beauty. Learning to be healthy is an ongoing process and there is not one formula that works for every body. Eating natural food without too many additives should be our highest priority.

We do not have to spend a lot of money on food. It also does not mean that we cannot enjoy a meal with friends who are on a different path. We have to find balance, a way that works for us. Often the simplest food, or temporarily eating nothing at all, may be best. Our overall habits and how we treat our body determines the way we feel and look. In the long run, our choices influence our relationship with others, and maybe even our finances. The food we eat may determine the places we frequent, the people we spend time with, the way we choose to spend our money, and overall preferences. People tend to think that diet has nothing to do with our wellbeing or that a healthy diet and eating organic food must be expensive. The alternative—being sick—is much more expensive. It not only costs money for doctors and prescriptions, but the time we lose could be used in more valuable ways. The pain and worry from being sick can be paralyzing, not to mention cause a loss of income.

Another concern are side effects. According to the American Medical Association more than 100,000 people in the US die from prescription drugs every year. Taking prescribed medicine—not the wrong medicine—has become the fourth leading cause of death in the United States. In order to stay healthy and prevent calamities it is important to make better food choices. Our body is a living miracle. It is built to clean and repair itself. Making the right choices, we can stay youthful and naturally beautiful till the last day of our lives. Eating can be one of the greatest pleasures, but it can also contribute to our downfall.

During my practice as a Nutritionist and yoga teacher, I have met people from three generations. I have seen tremendous changes for the better once people changed their diet. In fact, once we are in good health, we can feel ageless. What we eat or do not eat is important, but it is also important to stay physically and mentally active. It is important to always have something to look forward to, something that gives us joy. Being healthy, happy, and in love has nothing to do with age. It helps, however, to be in good shape to pursue our interests and find fulfillment in what we are doing. I love my work. It gives me an opportunity to meet some wonderful people. I also love to read, to dance, and travel, and I am always open to learning something new.

When my husband died unexpectedly in 2002, it was a tremendous blow for me. Only my work kept me going, but life goes on. Now I am in love again. The relationship motivates me to find the most effective, natural ways to slow down my own aging process and to enjoy life again. Love, more than any food, helps us to stay young, and happy people make a better world. Temporary challenges can be tough, but they can be a blessing in a sense that they motivate us to seek improvement. Nobody likes to suffer, and we have always choices. One of my teachers, John-Roger, used to say, "If you spill the milk, you can either sit and cry or you can wipe it up and move on with your life." Most of the time all that is required is to make a few simple changes. Are you ready?

Now is Our Greatest Opportunity

Most people work hard in pursuit of a better life, often forgetting to enjoy the present. Achieving better health is a stepping stone towards other areas of enjoyment and should be one of our priorities.

Next is perhaps the question of money. Money can do a lot of good if used wisely, and sometimes it takes worries off our mind. Money serves to buy goods. We also need shelter and transportation. We like to have friends. We like to love and be loved. Yet, time is more precious than all the other things, because without time we could not have the others. Time is our most valuable gift. A moment in time never comes back and our choices on how to use it determine the quality of our life. Wasting time in harmful actions is wasting the gift of life. Our thoughts, our words, and our present actions help us create the future we are looking for.

The wisdom of an unknown author describes how we can make the most of it. He says:

* Take time to think, it is the source of power.
* Take time to play, it is the secret of perpetual youth.
* Take time to read, it is the fountain of wisdom.
* Take time to pray, it is the greatest power on earth.

* Take time to love and be loved, it is a God-given privilege.
* Take time to be friendly, it is the road to happiness.
* Take time to laugh, it is the music of the soul.
* Take time to give, it is too short a day to be selfish.
* Take time to work, it is the price of success.
* Take time to do charity, it is the key to heaven.

We all want to feel good, to be healthy, wealthy and happy, and it is totally up to us how we use our time. It is never about waiting for something wonderful to happen in the future. Good things can happen soon if we start now, actively participating in our progress. Even small steps can make a difference. Sharing our blessings will bring more blessings to us. We can do it in simple ways by enjoying a meal together, telling a joke, letting people know we care, by listening to someone else's story, holding someone's hand, giving and receiving hugs, expressing appreciation, taking care of an animal, doing our work responsibly, or by enjoying our time with a loved one.

On occasion, it is good to spend time alone, sitting in silence, contemplating whatever we are grateful for, or simply loving and accepting ourselves no matter what. Each and every moment counts. Sometimes knowing that we are alive is enough. The more we are aware of our blessings, the richer our life will be, and the more we have to share.

Each day, each moment is a new opportunity, an opportunity to grow, to live, to love, and to share. Don't let it slip by. Use your time wisely. Time is our greatest gift, and it goes by faster than we think. When we get to the Pearly Gates, we may be asked what we did with our lives. Will the answer be, "I don't remember, time went by so fast. I just worked to make money. I divorced my spouse and won a lawsuit. I was sick and stressed out most of the time, so I hardly knew what was going on. I never helped anybody because nobody helped me either."

Or would you say, "I hugged my children, I took care of my mother. I kept my promises, I worked to earn a living. I enjoyed the little things. I taught something that might be useful to others. I watered the flowers. I walked in the park and swam in the ocean. I played with my children and groomed the dog. I praised God and took care of myself. I am thankful for life with all its ups and downs. I had opportunities to grow and to enjoy, and I always did the best I could."

Every day is an opportunity to create something better, to bring happiness to ourselves and others. Why waste time waiting to win the lottery? It might never happen. It is the little things that count, the things we do, the moments we enjoy that increase our wellbeing. Sharing whatever we have is another way to find happiness.

I love to spend time with my little dog Shanti. Like all animals, she is filled with unconditional love. I call her baby, even though she is already twelve years old. When I switch off the light in the evening, she comes running and cuddles up under the blankets with me. During the day, I watch her entertain herself with her toys. When she eats, she wags her tail with excitement. It is always the same dog food, but to her it seems to be the greatest delicacy. A little food, a little water, love, and shelter. How little it takes to create happiness! I love her, and she loves me, and we take care of each other.

For you, it might be your spouse, your children, or friends who give you pleasure by being around. Let them know how much you appreciate them. It is so important to take time, to care, to enjoy, to appreciate, including yourself. We never know if we have another opportunity. It is all part of life, part of being healthy and feeling good. Don't forget yourself! When you appreciate yourself, others will treat you with love and respect too. If you don't, nobody else will do it either. Be your own best friend. After all, you are the person you are going to spend the rest of your life with.

The time God gave us is our opportunity to create our life of choice. If we want abundance and prosperity, the best way to achieve it is by sharing. If you want more money, give money. If you want better health, sacrifice your appetite through occasional fasting. If you want more joy, bring joy to others. Time gives us opportunities.

In my teens, when I was in school in Germany, most of the students had a little album, where friends could write something memorable so we would never forget each other. Over the years, faces and names are long forgotten, but I still remember one of the most valuable entries. Somebody wrote in my album, "The joy we bring to others will return into our own heart." There is nothing better we can do with our time than to take care of ourselves and bring joy into the lives of others.

Whether we take care of ourselves, pray for ourselves or others, whether we praise somebody or give gifts, or whether we spend time with others, it is always a form of sharing our love, and this love will come back to us in some form. Our time and our love are the highest gifts available. Sharing them is a way to create the best life ever.

Sometimes it Takes Faith

Everything that happens to us, happens with our participation. We either create, promote or allow it, generally unintentionally, regardless of whether it is something we want or something we don't want. As soon as we take responsibility, there is a good chance our quality of life will improve. Blaming our parents, destiny, our partners, the Government or our luck in general, makes us victims. If we want a more positive outcome, we have to take responsibility and different action. We can always consult with others but eventually we reap what we set in motion. This applies to our state of health as well.

Disease does not come out of nowhere. Usually it is the result of a process that may have started years ago without us being aware of it or only with minor discomfort in the beginning. An unidentified author jokingly talks about how something so insignificant as taking an aspirin can eventually lead to major complications, including death. He calls it "**The American Death Ceremony**." He believes that on the average it takes about ten to fifteen years to complete the process, which is as follows: "When you have a headache, take an aspirin. If one is not enough, take another one. When two are not enough to get rid of the pain, use stronger compounds. Soon it will become necessary to add other medications for ulcers caused by the aspirin. After a few months, the new medication will disrupt your liver function or may affect your pancreas. If an infection develops, take antibiotics. They damage your red blood corpuscles, the spleen, and weaken your immune system. Now you have a good chance of needing more medication. All these chemicals will put such a strain on your kidneys that they should break down soon. It is time for cortisone and more antibiotics. They will destroy your natural resistance to disease altogether and you may expect a flare-up of all symptoms. When your kidneys are plugged up, you can keep going for awhile until there is such confusion in your body that nobody knows what to do and how they interact with each other. It does not matter. If you followed every step of the way, you are now ready for an appointment with your undertaker." This game is played by practically every American, except for a few ignorant souls who still follow Nature.

This sequence is supposed to be a funny exaggeration, but is it? So many people nowadays take medication for just about anything, prescribed or over the counter, without being aware of side effects or interactions with each other. It seems that those who "still follow Nature" remain stronger and last longer. Healthy people are the exception nowadays. Pain or discomfort signal that something is wrong, that we need to make changes. On the other hand, an absence of pain is not necessarily a sign of perfect health. There could be tooth loss, hair falling out, premature aging, skin conditions, hormone problems, being overweight or underweight, poor eyesight, low energy, or a number of other issues. They are all telling us that the body is not in optimum condition and that we need to and can do something about them.

When they don't feel well, most people go and see their physician. He or she orders tests and then comes up with a name for the ailment, called disease. There will always be something differing from the ideal values, because our body changes continuously due to the food we eat, our emotions and our thoughts. Nobody is in perfect health all the time but getting a label for our problem is usually not helpful, especially if it is serious, called incurable. Almost anything can be reversed once we eliminate its cause. Instead of giving us a label for a problem which we already know we have and medication with side effects to temporarily control the problem, it would be much more helpful to know the cause of the symptoms and learn how to eliminate it.

Our body is a miracle, and given the right care in time, it can completely heal itself. It may be sufficient to spend more time outdoors, to eat more fruit and vegetables, to avoid certain foods, to eat less frequently, or drink more water. Even taking a vacation might help. If your doctor told you that there is a good chance to get well without his help by making a few simple changes, you might be skeptical, although it is the truth. Besides, it is not in his best interest to do so. It is in **your** best interest to seek out alternatives without side effects. Educate yourself! Learn about health instead of reading about disease and its different symptoms.

Hearing the word "incurable" can almost paralyze people with fear, and instead of looking for alternatives first, they see traditional treatments as their only way out. There is a great number of people who choose to go the natural way and they not only managed to restore their health but they improved their quality of life along the way. One of them is a pretty nurse from Costa Rica. I had the good fortunate to meet her at a workshop, where she told me her story.

Ms. R. is a beautiful, lively woman with red hair, probably in her fifties, although she looks much younger. She used to work at a hospital in the section with terminally ill patients until she was diagnosed with cancer in her uterus. She was terrified because according to her observations most of the patients died after conventional treatments. She tried to ask one of the patients with the same problem as hers what she had done so far, because she wanted to skip those treatments, but the patient died before Ms. R. could get to her. She then started to look for alternatives.

After some research, she found a naturopathic clinic in Mexico. They recommended she eat only grapes and green leafy vegetables. During that time, Ms. R. said she eliminated a lot of nasty, greenish stuff through her vagina. She described it as something that looked like honeycomb. She also experienced considerable weight loss due to the toxins she eliminated. After six weeks, she went back to see her gynecologist, who examined her and told her that her uterus was as healthy as that of a woman in her twenties. At the time, Ms. R. was already a grandmother. The diet not only healed her, it rejuvenated her whole body. Nobody would have guessed her age. She looked like thirty-five, but had a daughter in her thirties.

In most cases, detoxification is enough to start the body's self-healing. The result may be more bowel movements, elimination through the urine causing unusual smell or cloudiness, skin eruptions, tiredness or drastic weight loss. Once elimination is activated, we might feel worse in the beginning. We are not getting sicker. We are getting healthy. The bad stuff is trying to find its way out. Most of the time to see results requires consistency. Afterwards the white of our eyes may become clearer, our complexion rosier, body odor disappears, and we may find ourselves more energized and in a better mood. We may even feel and look rejuvenated.

Whether we go the traditional way or choose natural alternatives, there is no guarantee of success either way. The difference may be that your quality of life may be better after you overcome a problem naturally. Such was the case with many people who at one time suffered from something called "incurable" and then went a different route and eventually became teachers to others.

First a Student, Then a Teacher

Buddha taught that all human beings have two things in common: They want to be happy and they want to avoid pain. Most people live in the illusion that working longer hours and making more money will bring them happiness once they are able to buy the things they have been dreaming of. Those things can make us happy for a little while but they do not fulfill us in the long run. We like the new car, the better home, a raise in pay. It is great to pass an exam, to find a mate, or celebrate the next birthday. Once we achieve these goals, the excitement goes away and so does the "happiness", and we look for new goals. It is like climbing a mountain before we go into another valley and then look for a higher top, which may be a better car, a bigger house, or a new partner. And then we start all over again.

Good health is so important because it is the basis to enjoy other things. Sometimes we feel sorry for people who do not have certain commodities, and yet they may be happier than we are. Living near the Mexican border, I often see "poor" Tarahumara Indians. Occasionally they walk for miles to get food. A little rice, a handful of beans, a few coins make them happy. Regardless of their material lack, they seem to be in the best of health and most of them have a friendly smile on their faces. Just living in the moment without worrying can bring great joy. If we choose to, we can be happy watching the sun rise, feeling the air on our skin, having food in our stomach, giving and receiving hugs, and above all, being grateful for what we do have.

To take care of ourselves is something that should not be complicated. When we are young, we take life for granted. We eat and drink whatever appeals to us, go to parties, pop a few pills, or in some cases take drugs to get high. As time goes by, we may gain weight, feel sluggish, cannot sleep anymore, or are diagnosed with some kind of illness. Few people take care of themselves before problems show up. The good thing is our body is forgiving and most symptoms can be reversed.

Unless it is something serious or there is an emergency, natural remedies will be of great help. Through experience we can learn what works for us and what does not. One gentleman used to get two or three colds a month in winter. Once he started taking garlic and lemon juice instead of over the counter drugs, he strengthened his immune system and was hardly ever bothered by another cold again. There are always choices. Do we want to fight disease or build health? They might look the same, but actually they are opposites to each other.

One of the simplest ways to increase our wellbeing is through the food we eat. Our body is like a computer—it reacts to whatever we put in it. The consequences might not show up immediately and often seem totally unrelated. It can take years before the body reacts, like in the case of tooth decay. We may have forgotten that years ago we ate all those candies, took antibiotics, or controlled a headache with medication. The body never forgets! Disease does not come out of nowhere. We created it, and just as we create disease we can also create health.

One of the most famous teachers in the field of natural healing was Professor Arnold Ehret (1866-1922), a pioneer in fasting and inner cleansing. He is the author of several books, including *The Mucusless Diet Healing System* and *Radical*

Fasting. At the age of thirty-one, he was diagnosed with Bright's Disease, suffered from kidney trouble and consumption. He was declared incurable. First, he tried "fortifying" diets at prestigious clinics and experienced temporary improvement. However, it was not until he came up with his famous mucusless diet, consisting mainly of fruit, vegetables, and occasional fasting that he became an image of health and beauty.

He recommends avoiding starchy foods like bread and pasta as well as all dairy products. He demonstrated the effectiveness of this diet when after a seven day fast he traveled with a friend through Northern Italy walking continuously for fifty-six hours without rest, sleep, or food. Both men drank only water. Afterwards, they continued eating only one vegetarian meal a day consisting of fruit. At some point, they met people infected with cholera. Although the disease is highly contagious and caused many deaths at the time, they never caught it. Their blood was so clean, they had become immune, proving that disease can only exist in a toxic body.

Recently I met a lady who had suffered for years from diabetes and high blood pressure. She is perfectly healthy now. She told me that for a little over a month she has been on a vegan diet. No cheese, no eggs, no fish, and she never felt better. Her daughter, who had Lupus, started the idea of eating mainly fruit and vegetables, and she is doing well too. They are both practically on a mucusless diet as Arnold Ehret recommended after tracing his own "incurable" Bright's disease back to eating starchy food and then healed himself simply by changing his diet.

Sickness is the body's effort to free itself from toxins. The body tries to eliminate what should not be there and brings it to the surface. It may present itself as a cold, a fever, skin rashes, hair falling out, swelling, bloating, extreme tiredness or other symptoms. Instead of fighting these symptoms, we need to support the natural cleaning action. The body talks to us, either through wellbeing or what we call "disease." There may be pain, bad smell, digestive troubles, weight problems, high cholesterol, insomnia, discharges, irregular heartbeat, loss of appetite, headaches, protruding veins, or other symptoms. When we see a doctor to get rid of these symptoms, he takes some tests and then prescribes medication. The medication might stop the discomfort, but it does not get rid of the cause. Therefore, no permanent healing can take place. Medication adds more toxins to the ones that are already present and produces other side effects.

The main cause for most disease is toxic matter, often accumulated over time. Deficiencies may be caused by toxins as well, because it is not the food we ingest that counts, but rather the nutrients we absorb. Toxic matter in our body can be the cause of parasites, mold and fungus, including Candidiasis, which all prevent proper absorption of nutrients and can be the cause of serious illness, including cancer.

Sometimes it seems like a miracle when all the unwanted symptoms disappear. If it is a miracle, we created it. There is no way we can be well when we eat junk food, lead a sedentary lifestyle, or have negative emotions. It is hard to feel good when we hate ourselves, our job, and almost everybody around us. Taking a walk outdoors and breathing fresh air can already make a difference. Living within our means can reduce excess worrying. Reading the Scriptures may bring more peace of mind, and skipping a meal gives our digestive system a temporary rest. Diet foods, on the other hand, are among the worst offenders, not to mention the use of microwave ovens, and both ought to be avoided. Inner cleansing and strengthening the immune system will take care of more than 80% of all health challenges, regardless of their definition.

If somebody says there is no cure for a problem, all it means is that the person telling you so has not found one. If medical doctors had all the answers, they would be the healthiest people on the planet. Apparently, just the opposite is true.

Dr. Joel Wallach on his famous, humorous tape "Dead doctors do not lie" says that the average age for doctors is under sixty. Dr. Wallach is a Naturopathic Doctor, a Veterinarian, and also has a degree in allopathic medicine. Although he is married to a physician, he believes very much in natural healing and stresses the importance of minerals and healthy fats in our diet. I met him when he was over seventy and still looked young. He is a dynamic, extremely knowledgeable speaker. He has his own hair color and no age spots. Jokingly, he said that his formula to staying healthy was that whenever he has a problem, he first asks his doctor wife what to do and then does the opposite of what she recommends. Dr. Wallach teaches what he preaches, which is mainly to ingest more minerals. Our soils today are depleted of minerals and, therefore, our food does not have the nutrients it used to have.

All medication has side effects, sometimes serious ones. Pharmaceutical companies are required to disclose them, although most likely they prefer people would not to know about them. Just by watching the commercials on TV, you may learn about some of the dangers. Some products can cause nausea, dizziness, vomiting, loss of hearing, palpitations, internal bleeding, headaches, breathing problems, and sometimes even death. Many times, products have been recalled after hundreds of people already died or suffered other serious consequences. I am surprised that some men still buy the little blue pill for sexual performance. A sexual problem is a health problem. Once we eliminate the cause, men will have no problems in the bedroom, at least as far as performance is concerned. Although men are advised to call their doctor if they experience a sudden loss of hearing and eyesight, I doubt your busy doctor will be sitting there waiting for a call. Besides, how are you going to dial his number when you lost your eyesight and your hearing? Herbs, vitamins, and diets are effective and have never killed anyone.

Years back, there was a true story on television about a man who healed himself of cancer. It was explained as an unexpected remission. When officially there is no known cure, one can only speak of "remission" or say that the person has been misdiagnosed. The gentleman in question had been diagnosed with terminal cancer and was given a life expectancy of about three months. His doctors suggested he undergo radiation and chemotherapy. The patient inquired about his chances of survival after treatment, and was told there was no guarantee, maybe six months. The doctors would do whatever they could. The best they could hope for was that maybe he would live six months instead of three. He thanked his physicians and instead of submitting himself to the treatments they suggested, he decided to live whatever time he had left in the best possible way. He took a vacation. I think he said he went on a cruise. He drank cognac, the best of its kind. He smoked cigars, the most expensive ones. After all, he wanted to have a nice memory of his stay on earth. He enjoyed himself as best as he could during what he believed were his last days.

After three months, the time his doctors had estimated he would die without their treatment, he went back for a check-up and lo and behold, there was no trace of cancer! They could not believe it. The man looked happier and healthier than ever, and said he never felt better. Was it because he accepted his situation? Was it because the stress was gone? Was it the fresh air or the cognac? Nobody knows. The fact is, he did something different and is now looking forward to a new life.

Dr. John Christopher (1909-1983) is still known today as a famous herbalist. In his teens, he suffered from hardening of the arteries due to rheumatoid arthritis, which affected his heart. He was told that he was lucky if he made it to his twenties. He returned to health with a vegetarian diet consisting mainly of fruit, vegetables, grains and nuts in combination with inner cleansing and occasional fasting. Later on, he studied the effects of herbs and his favorite was cayenne pepper, of which he took large amounts daily. Cayenne pepper is believed to unclog the arteries similar to a roto-rooter. He became a Master Herbalist and world-famous teacher. Dr. Christopher outlived all his physicians who had given him only a few years to live, and was in excellent health when he died at the age of seventy-four in a car accident.

Another outstanding example of vibrant health and youthfulness was Dr. Otoman Zar-Adusht Ha'nish (1844-1936). In his time, he was one of the greatest spiritual leaders. Not much is known about his origin. At the age of three, he was abandoned in a monastery in Tibet, where he learned and practiced many of the disciplines unknown in the Western world. He studied the teachings of Zarathustra and became the founder of the Mazdaznan Healing System, which has something to do with light and colors with regard to the food we eat. He enjoyed recognition as a physician, scientist, artist, inventor, as well as founder of several spiritual, religious and ethics movements.

Students of Mazdaznan follow a vegetarian diet and choose their food according to its color and in accordance with their physical constitution. The basics are determined by the measurements of the scull, known as phrenology, and they can either be predominantly physical, spiritual, or intellectual. People with a physical constitution tend to have a round face and should prefer food with the color red, which strengthens the liver and improves circulation. People with an intellectual inclination and a more oval shaped face benefit more from a diet with at least 50% yellow food, like nuts, grains, and oils, which benefit their glandular system. Those who are spiritually inclined benefit the most from food with blue undertones. This includes green, leafy vegetables, thereby increasing the absorption of iron and oxygen. For them, choosing green apples over red ones would be more beneficial. The same applies to grapes and other fruit. Legumes, beans, and rice are recommended for all.

Dr. O. Ha'nish fasted many times for forty days or more, and at the age of sixty did not look older than twenty-five. A photograph taken of him at that age shows him with a full head of hair in his own color and youthful skin without wrinkles or blemishes. In his nineties, a few years before his death, he was still in excellent shape, walking tall and straight.

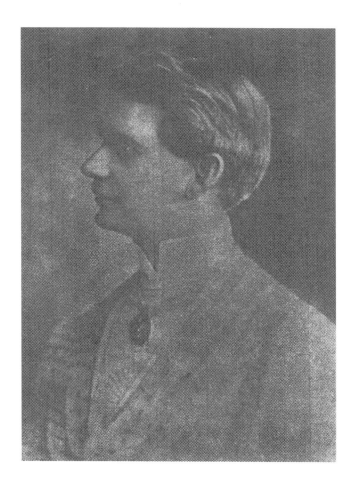

Photograph of Dr. O'Hanish
when he was sixty years of age.
He fasted many times forty days and more.

These are some of the world-famous healers who gave guidance to others. Today, there are hundreds of people who have learned to overcome disease naturally and became teachers. Among the most famous ones in the United States are David Wolfe, Markus Rothkranz, Victoria Boutenko, and the beautiful Tonya Zavasta, author of *Beauty for Raw* and *Quantum Eating*. All of them are raw-foodists and recommend a mineral and enzyme rich diet. Markus Rothkranz looks younger at fifty-four than he did at twenty-five.

Natural methods are timeless and can be practiced in the privacy of your own home at a low cost. By taking care of ourselves naturally, we can prevent and correct almost any disease. Conventional treatments often cause damage to the immune system. Although the U.S. has very advanced medical technology, it ranks extremely low in health statistics. Besides, medical errors and procedures are the third leading cause of death in the country after cancer and heart attacks. Prevention is always best. Once we learn how to take care of ourselves naturally, we can create our own miracles.

Mother Nature's Ways

Over the years, I have seen people in desperate situations, suffering physically, emotionally, mentally, financially, and socially. Often, their health challenges were at the root of the other problems. Some were unable to work and had spent most of their money and hopes on medications that did more harm than good. Others had been abandoned by their life partners due to their illness, and again others passed on to a better life after times of agony. Maybe I feel such deep empathy with them, because there was a time when I was in a similar situation—desperate, and wondering why it happened to me.

Although I grew up in times of scarcity after World War II in Germany, as a child and young woman I had been in good health. Looking back, I attribute my good health to the fact that I spent most of my childhood in my grandfather's garden, living on fruit, potatoes, corn, and a few other vegetables the garden produced. We had five chickens, and the only meat I saw in those times was when one of the chickens disappeared and we had chicken soup afterwards.

After finishing high school, I went to study in London to become an interpreter. Of course, I had very little money and often lived on candies and the junk food I could afford. Whenever I got sick, I took medication to get over the problem as soon as possible. Gradually, I lost my good health. In 1965,

I immigrated to Mexico. Soon I suffered from nausea, irregular bleeding, profuse hair loss, temporary deafness, skin disorders and other issues. I saw different specialists, praying each time that the next one would be the one to help me. Was it the altitude, the unaccustomed heat, the different food? I never knew, and in spite of all the prescription medication, which included antibiotics, hormones, vitamins, protein diets, rubbing my scalp with ammonia, and other procedures, I did not get better. In hindsight, I realize that it was part of God's plan for me. Suffering often leads to the greatest turning points in our lives. If it had not been for my own desperate situation with apparently no way out, I would never have discovered the blessings of nutrition and inner cleansing. I also learned to understand the suffering of others and later on help them even when everything else had failed.

As far as I remember, it all started with a blessing in disguise: After not getting any better with medical treatments, one day I collapsed in a street in Mexico City. It was not from exhaustion, nor from the smog in the air, or some kind of emotional stress. I was only in my early twenties and could take a certain amount of adversity. Apparently, it was caused by something else. We create our problems, unwillingly and unknowingly, and this was no exception.

Years prior to the crisis, I had been eating fast food in cheap restaurants and tried to appease my appetite with candy bars. It saved money and time, both of which I had very little as a student. When I did not feel well, I took over-the-counter drugs, antibiotics, quinine, vitamins, hormones and whatever I was told would help, and also because I could not afford to miss time at work and school. Then there was dental work, amalgam fillings, X-rays, and prescribed medication for the ever-increasing symptoms. My skin started breaking out and no amount of cleansing could get rid of the severe acne. I started suffering from headaches that got more and more severe, bleeding in between my periods, unbearable cramps, liver pains, constipation, endometriosis, bloating, and profuse hair loss.

At first, I saw general practitioners, then different specialists who sincerely tried to help me. It was one physician after another, more and more medication, more specialists and then time spent in the hospital. Instead of seeing an improvement, new symptoms appeared, and eventually I had to spend most of my Saturdays and Sundays in the outpatient section of the general hospital. My hair loss became so advanced that I could see my scalp in daylight. I hardly dared to touch or comb my hair, because I could not stand to see it coming out by the handfuls. I would have done anything to stop it. What prospects did I have of ever leading a normal life or finding a decent job, much less a husband, after all these years of study?

No matter what I tried, and how many specialists I saw, my condition did not get better. Some doctors diagnosed me with liver disease, others said it was hormone related, the dermatologist recommended I rub my head with ammonia. Then they prescribed something for the kidneys and antibiotics. The gynecologist gave me hormones and Vitamin B injections. Severe acne showed up and the more I washed my face, the worse it got. At a time, it was over 250 hairs a day and all I could do was just sit there and cry.

In my agony, I started reading books on diseases. Of course, I was no medical expert, but somebody had to find a cure! Why not me? Nobody seemed to have a clue as to what was wrong with me and why my body did not respond favorably to any of the treatments. In fact, the intermittent bleedings between my periods and skin rashes got worse, my hair kept falling out, my headaches and cramps became more frequent and seemed unbearable at times. Eventually, I was convinced I had gonorrhea and insisted on having my blood tested for it. The tests came back negative. I insisted that they must be wrong, because I had all the symptoms of this terrible disease. I even got mad at the doctor, because he refused to treat me for gonorrhea, the main reason being that I did not have it. I was not convinced. I was desperate. Nobody had come up with a real diagnosis or something that brought relief.

The thought of being unable to support myself in a competitive world was frightening. I kept looking for answers. How did I get these problems? What had caused them? There was no particular label for my "disease" and obviously no cure. As time went by, I felt more and more desperate. What do you do when you get to that point? You cry out to God for help, and that was what I did. If somebody had told me to rub skunk oil on my scalp and eat bats' waste, I would have done it. Fortunately, that was not necessary.

Looking back, I firmly believe that no prayer remains without answer. One day, somebody mentioned a healer, a German naturopathic doctor who had come to Mexico years ago. He had studied the herbs of the country and used no drugs, just diets, natural herb teas and tonics. People spoke of him with great reverence because of the many miraculous healings he had achieved. They reported that he had cured them even after everything else had failed. As soon as I heard of him, I was convinced that he must be the answer to my prayers. If anybody could do miracles, it had to be him. And that was exactly what I expected: A miracle.

I went to see this healer after work. He gave his consultations in a poor neighborhood and his fees were reasonable. He had no diplomas that identified him as a medical doctor. In fact, he was not a medical doctor. His original profession had been in the airline business. Nobody knew for sure. Somebody mentioned he came from a long line of vegetarians. Everything about him was kind of unusual: He did not have a telephone and was not listed in the phone book. One could not make an appointment. To see him, one had to stand in line certain days of the week and wait for one's turn, sometimes for hours. Rich or poor, high and mighty or not, there were no exceptions. We all had to wait. My major concern was my hair loss, since all the other problems were not visible to the eyes. I was wondering what else I should mention so he could make an accurate diagnostic. Little did I understand that **everything** in the body originates inside, and there is no need to specify the individual problems, like doctors do. All problems depend on what is going on inside. Even a beauty problem is a health problem! So is a weight problem, a skin problem, a hair problem, an energy problem, and everything else.

When my turn came to see this unusual man, Dr. Juan Sperl, or Don Juanito as he was lovingly called by the Mexican people, I was surprised by his gentleness and extreme simplicity. Although he was in his eighties, he was elegantly dressed in a light-colored suit and he had an air of youthfulness about him. He was tall and slim and still had blond hair. Apparently, he liked to smoke. All the flowerpots were full of cigarette stubs, with no ashtrays in sight. Although he had already seen more than seventy people on that particular day, he showed no signs of fatigue.

His "office" consisted of a table and three old chairs on a patio: one for himself, one for the secretary, who took notes, and the third for the patient. No telephone, no filing cabinets, no complicated instruments in the room. Sterilization seemed to be a word unheard of in this place. There were bugs crawling around the potted plants, cracks in the walls (probably from a previous earthquake) and tiny lizards running across the room. The floor looked clean, although it was hard to tell whether it had been swept recently or not. Once in a while, a cat stopped by and meowed, probably looking for mice and lizards. Definitely, it was quite different from doctors' offices in my native Germany. But what did I care? All I wanted was to get my health back.

To my disappointment, and in contrast to all the other specialists I had seen before, Dr. Sperl did not ask one single question. I think he did not even ask my name. With a friendly smile on his face and a magnifying glass in his hand, he approached me and examined the iris of my eyes. As I learned later on, this evaluation is called "iridology" and shows the state of the entire body. He did not have to ask. He could see. The irises truthfully reflect the condition of different organs, the blood, the nervous system, toxic matter, deficiencies, and so much more. Once the causes are taken care of, the symptoms will disappear. There is no need to attach a name to the "disease."

Dr. Sperl only said "Hmmm" to me after studying my iris for a moment and then mumbled something to the secretary. She took notes and handed me a sheet with his recommendations for a change in my diet and some herbs. I was anxious to know more. What had he seen in my eyes? How long would it take until I would see results?

Dr. Sperl said, "Come back in four weeks!" and that was it. My "prescription" consisted of dietary guidelines, drinking specific herbal teas, days of semi-fasting or eating only one kind of fruit, and cold-water compresses around the stomach area. No drugs. No shots. No prescriptions. And yet, this very first program he gave me was so powerful that in less than two months it turned my health around, and eighty percent of all my symptoms disappeared. In two months, I felt like a new person.

The fee I paid for my first consultation in naturopathic medicine was fifty pesos or the equivalent to four dollars at the time, which even then was a moderate amount. I followed the indications to the T. After all, I did not want to lose more hair, and this German doctor was my last hope. The third week on his program I felt so good that I decided to continue a little longer than the recommended four weeks, just to make sure this newly acquired sense of well-being was real and not part of my imagination.

I followed the program for a full two months before I went back, feeling wonderful. The night before my appointment I could hardly sleep. I was so excited. In my mind, I prepared a speech of gratitude. I could have kissed this man. He had given me my life back! And all for four dollars, plus the price of the herbs.

When my turn came to see him, I could hardly utter a word. I was overwhelmed, and also very shy. Tears came to my eyes and instead of the speech I had prepared the night before, all I could say was, "Thank you, doctor!" With the simplicity and humbleness that characterized this great man, he smiled and responded with words I will never forget: "**Don't thank me. It is Mother Nature who does the healing. We only have to give Her a hand**."

Nobody could have expressed it better! He changed my life forever. Nature **never** fails, but we have to do our part. After my own success, especially after everything else I had tried before had so utterly failed, I studied as much as I could about natural healing. After all, I had enough problems in my own body to learn from. Dr. Sperl taught me many practical lessons, and up to this day I consider him to be one of the greatest healers that has ever lived. As he so modestly put it, it was not him who did the healing. It was Mother Nature, but we all know that God sends His servants.

Dr. Juan Sperl's Miracle Diet

By now you may be curious about Dr. Sperl's miraculous diet, since it has helped not only me, but thousands of others achieve radiant health. If you are willing to try it, it will probably do the same for you. He never called the program miraculous. He was too modest to do so. However, the results people from all walks of life achieved with it, including some "important" people, were so amazing that the Mexican government conferred to him the title of Dr. Honor is Causa and he became Dr. Juan Sperl, although he never set foot in a medical school. Even today some of the most prestigious naturopathic healers, clinics, and nutritionists use part of his program with excellent results. Key to its success is probably the overall alkalizing effect of a vegetarian diet with lots of raw fruit and vegetables, combined with periodic fasting.

When I met Dr. Sperl, he was around eighty-six years old. His goal was to alleviate people's suffering by teaching them to eat differently, and eliminate disease without costly and invasive procedures. Sometimes he saw close to 100 people a day and never seemed to get tired. Coming originally from a vegetarian family in Germany, he became one of the most famous healers in Mexico. He married an Indian woman from the State of Veracruz. Through her, he acquired a profound knowledge of native herbs and learned to prepare his own mixtures and tinctures. It was a valuable asset to his healing, because even today Mexican herbs are considered to be most effective, especially those coming from the Tarahuamara Indians.

Dr. Sperl learned to relate the signs in a person's eyes to their state of health and his "diagnosis" usually proved accurate. Today, iridology is applied by naturopaths all over the world. Among his clients were medical doctors, politicians, famous artists, and ordinary people. The healings were amazing. The wife of a medical doctor, who was already in menopause, managed to fulfill her life's dream and conceive a healthy baby. People with arthritis started to walk again. Others saved their eyesight and healed themselves of diabetes, cancer, and other illnesses after being given up on by the medical community. He was a true healer of the people, and he was affordable. People loved him, usually referring to him as Don Juanito.

Although his expertise seemed like magic at the time, today there are several schools that teach nutrition, iridology, and herbology. Iridology, in particular, is a valuable asset, since it shows the condition of organs, the blood, the nervous system, as well as toxic matter and residues of pharmaceutical medication in the body. Just by observing a person's irises, with the help of a magnifying glass, it is possible for the trained practitioner to see the condition of the entire body. Healthy areas of the iris have no signs. Another advantage of iridology is that it is completely non-invasive. No X-rays and no blood tests are required.

As far as I can tell, Dr. Sperl's diet was similar for all patients. Of course, the sicker a person, the stricter the diet has to be, because there is more urgency for recovery. His program activates the self-healing power in each person. It also helps to reach our ideal weight and has rejuvenating effects. The longer you follow the program, the greater the benefits.

Dr. Sperl believed in fasting. Generally, he was in very good health. His consultations were held in a poor neighborhood and he used to travel by bus from his home to the "office". If you ever traveled by bus in Mexico City in those times, you will understand that this can be a hazardous undertaking. During the main traffic hours, the buses were so crowded that some passengers hung out of the windows and doors. The younger ones, mainly students, sat on the roof. Inside the bus, people were pushing against each other, surrounded by skillful pick pockets who made their living on public transport. As a result, Dr. Sperl got pushed off the bus several times and suffered severe injuries, where he had to be taken to the hospital. The doctors were always amazed at his speedy recovery.

On one occasion, one of the assisting physicians could not contain his curiosity and directly asked him if he had a secret. Although he was already in his eighties, every time his injuries healed at a speed that only happens in a young person. The secret was in his blood. Dr. Sperl smiled and replied that it must be his diet. I do not think he followed any particular diet. He also was a heavy smoker, of which hundreds of cigarette stubs in the flower pots gave testimonial. And yet, there was a cause for his rejuvenation. The secret had indeed to do with his diet: Every year, around May, when mangoes are in season, Dr. Sperl fasted for forty days eating nothing but mangoes. Apparently, this diet purified his blood and kept him young until the day he died. He still worked when he was in his nineties.

Looking back, I can only say that I never felt so good as when I followed Dr. Sperl's diet and the best compliment came from our family doctor in Germany. After examining me and finding me in the best state of health ever, he asked what I had been doing. I told him about the diet, but he did not believe it. Eating fruit only every fourth day to improve one's health was against everything he had learned in medical school. Today, research in anti-aging medicine has proven that intermittent fasting is the safest way to lose weight, stay healthy, and slow down the aging process. Here are the recommendations from the miracle diet as I remember them:

1) Follow a vegetarian diet. Dr. Sperl did allow eggs and dairy products.
2) For a whole month begin breakfast, lunch and dinner with the same kind of fruit. It could be a pear, an apple, strawberries, papaya, prunes or pineapple. Since all fruits have different effects, he chose the fruit carefully for each patient.
3) He added an herbal tea according to individual needs. Today, you can get herbal mixtures at health food stores.
4) The heart of the program was a salad consisting of watercress, celery, parsley, lettuce and onion. Other raw veggies or herbs could be added for taste. In vegetarian restaurants sometimes spinach, tomatoes, cilantro, carrots, cooked beets, sprouts, almonds, olives, or avocado are added. Even fruit like papaya, slices of apple or pear, can be included.
5) The salad was to be accompanied by a glass of fresh carrot or tomato juice. Both are full of vitamins, minerals, and enzymes. Some people have problems with their teeth, and instead of chewing the salad may want to convert the ingredients into a green smoothie.
6) Between meals one would either sip water, grapefruit juice when appropriate, or tamarind water. Sometimes Dr. Sperl recommended a glass of water with a tablespoonful of apple cider vinegar and raw honey.

I remember that I ate three full meals a day and still dropped to about 86 pounds. I was so skinny that even I was wondering where I was going with this diet, hoping every month to regain the lost pounds. I had started at 110 or 112 pounds. I had not been overweight, but I was very sick and full of toxins. My collarbone started sticking out and my knees looked like those of a horse. My boyfriend threatened to stop talking to me if I stayed on the program. The only thing that kept me going was that I felt very good and hoped this was only a temporary side effect.

Although I was anxious to gain weight and ate as much as I could, I still got skinnier every month. Dr. Sperl explained to me that the body was cleansing itself and would not stop doing so until the blood was free of toxins. Only then would the body return to health regardless of the amount of food I ate. Another reason for my weight loss and speedy recovery was that I misunderstood the instructions. My Spanish was not very good at the time and instead of eating the salad once a day "before my meal" I ate it before breakfast, lunch, and dinner. It was not my favorite food, but I started feeling better day by day and I knew that my alternative was to stay sick. It was a misunderstanding, and one salad a day would have been enough. People who are overweight might want to try eating more salads with green, leafy vegetables to speed up their weight loss and improve their health at the same time.

All of Dr. Sperl's patients were advised to live exclusively on one kind of fruit every fourth day, alternating with chamomile tea. The amount of fruit did not matter, as long as it was one kind only. This kind of fasting or semi-fasting is particularly effective due to the amount of fiber, vitamins, minerals, and natural water contained in the fruit. People sometimes complain about headaches, loose stools, stomach cramps, painful gas, a coated tongue, bad breath or headaches when on this mono-diet and think they are getting sicker instead of better. I remember having all of them, but my energy returned. This kind of diet brings toxins to the surface and can be compared to a powerful housecleaning.

You might see worms, mucus, black or green stuff in the toilet. This is what is keeping you sick. It is not the nasty stuff that is coming out of the body that is bad; the danger is when it stays inside and does **not** come out. It is the cause of all disease! Another way to accelerate the internal cleansing is with enemas or colonics. Words do not describe how clean you feel afterwards. The average person is believed to have about five to ten pounds of waste in their colon. Such internal putrefaction creates foul smelling gas, lots of acidity in the bloodstream, and is a breeding ground for undesirable microorganisms, virus, and fungus.

Another important detail of Dr. Sperl's program was the cold wrap. It is a wrap you use at night that activates elimination and calms the nervous system. It helps you sleep better, corrects constipation, gas, water retention, high blood pressure, or can be used to lower a fever. Sometimes, midwives recommend it after childbirth to help mama get her waistline back.

Here is how to use it: Before you go to bed at night you take a piece of cotton muslin (as thick as you can get it), about half a yard wide and approximately two yards long, depending on your body circumference. Fold it lengthwise in half, then dip it into cold water and wring it out. You can leave it in the refrigerator before use. It has to be cold. Otherwise, it has no effect. Before going to bed, you wrap the muslin tightly around your body from the waist down. Start wrapping on your right side, go across the abdomen, then across the back to your right hip and again across the abdomen at your left hip. The muslin is then covered with a dry towel and tied up with a string, belt, or underwear to hold it in place. It is important to keep it tight and it will warm up immediately. During their menstrual period, women are advised not to use the cold wrap because it might produce cramps.

In the morning, you take the wrap off, rinse out all the toxins, and then use it again at night. If people have taken medication or are heavy smokers, the muslin will get stained or smell bad.

Small Steps, Sure Results

Today, there are many effective natural programs out there, some of them similar to Dr. Sperl's diet. If you are on medication, you cannot leave it overnight. Doing so could be dangerous. Ask your physician before you make any changes. All you can do is wean yourself off gradually with your doctor's help.

It is ideal to feel good all the time, to have good eyesight, good hearing, good memory, be flexible, neither be overweight nor too skinny. We want to have clear skin, shiny hair, and be in a good mood. In other words, we want to enjoy life without impediments. In case of a check-up our blood pressure, blood sugar, cholesterol and whatever else the doctor is measuring should be within normal ranges. We like to sleep well at night, be sexually adequate, and be able to enjoy life. Good health can be achieved by making a few changes and then follow them consistently. So many people have been successful in overcoming difficulties, and so can we. I am always surprised to find that some of the healthiest, wealthiest, nicest, most beautiful people are actually very simple. They all started somewhere and often it were their very problems that motivated them to search for alternatives and go a different route. The only thing we have to know is that it can be done.

Basically, all natural healing is about internal cleansing and detoxification, as well as choosing the right nutrients. This combination builds up the immune system. Some healers believe in partial fasting or mono-diets with fruit or green juices. Even eating brown rice for a whole day or drinking bone broth increases your chances of improvement. Most programs include healthier eating in combination with exercise. It might be a good idea to get a notebook and write things down when you start and track your progress, which could be how much you weigh, what issues are bothering you, what your goals are, and the progress you are making.

Since it requires some discipline, you could make your own plan in advance and, as an example, commit to a daily walk of fifteen minutes outdoors. Or you may commit to eating only fruit for breakfast for a whole month. If it is easier, skip dinner. The choices are infinite. As you commit to something and take action, write down if it helped you and check on your progress once a week.

If your time and budget allow it, you may want to go to a place where you have the guidance and supervision of experts. This is where you learn the most. You practice and learn at the same time. You will also find likeminded people who like to share their experiences. Some come for health issues, others want to rejuvenate. Most of these places offer classes and lectures as part of their program. The idea is not about temporarily eating certain foods and then going back to old habits. It is about learning to create a better life. Once you see the changes in others with your own eyes and get your own experiences, most likely you will keep up part of the program and gradually feel better.

There is a difference between medical procedures and natural healing. The first gets rid of symptoms. Natural healing benefits everybody. It increases health and beauty, whether you start out sick or do it preventatively. Inner cleansing brings toxic matter to the surface and then helps the body to heal on its own. All healing is done by the body itself, strengthening your own immune system. Health and beauty start on the inside.

Many of the great teachers, like Paul Bragg, Dr. Sperl and others, recommend fasting or semi-fasting as the ultimate resource. Paul Bragg, famous author and pioneer in the field of natural healing, used to fast four times every year for at least one week and he was still active in his nineties. Dr. Sperl maintained his youthfulness with his yearly forty-day mango diet, which kept him in excellent condition till the day he died, still working and seeing patients in his nineties. But before we get to any kind of fasting, we want to start with something simpler. A journey of a thousand miles starts with the first step.

A good start for anyone may be to eat more natural, organic food. It could be to read books on health, spend time in nature or with family, taking a vacation, taking up a hobby, or simply watching less television. Life is the greatest gift. Enjoy it. If you want to make changes, the most important thing is to get started, and here are a few suggestions:

1) First thing in the morning drink a glass of water with the juice of one lime or lemon to flush out toxins. The Spanish raw-food expert Nicolas Capó claimed that lemons help to heal over 160 different ailments. Used regularly, they help to avoid many kinds of illness. Of course, Mr. Capo recommended more than one lemon a day for his cures, but the juice of just one lemon in a glass of water every day will already make a difference.

2) Once a day, either before lunch or dinner, eat a salad with fresh greens. Pasta "salad" with cheese is not a salad! Greens have fiber, chlorophyll, minerals, vitamins, and enzymes. The color green being the most predominant one in nature is also the most healing one for the heart, the nervous system, and for the digestive tract. We know that large animals like the cow, the ox, the elephant and the giraffe live on grass and leaves, and form a strong,

beautiful, perfectly healthy body. It is not true that we need to eat large amounts of protein to be strong. In fact, one of the strongest and most beautiful men of our time is Dr. Amen-Ra, a world champion in heavy weight lifting and life extension specialist. He eats only one vegan meal a day with less than 1500 calories and has a special shake with his own secret ingredients.

In case you have problems chewing, you can enjoy a smoothie instead of the salad, blending fresh greens like spinach, parsley, kale, cucumbers or others, with fruit for better taste. The chlorophyll deodorizes and alkalizes the body and keeps our breath fresh. Greens are an ideal supplement and should not be missing in any diet unless you are on blood thinning medication and need to avoid anything with Vitamin K in it, especially greens.

3) Just as important as dietary improvement is exercise. The best exercise is walking. At least fifteen minutes in the morning or in the evening will cheer you up. Never walk in the heat of the sun, since this will deplete your energy instead of adding to it. Diet cannot replace exercise. The Swedish philosopher Soren Kierkegaard said, "Above all, do not lose your desire to walk. Every day I walk myself into a state of wellbeing and walk away from every illness. I have walked myself into my best thoughts, and I know of no thought so burdensome that one cannot walk away from."

Walking brings oxygen to your blood. It clears the mind, reduces stress. It improves digestion and improves our circulation. It helps shape our body and accelerates weight loss. It might help let go of old grudges and forgive any wrongs done to you, and see life in a whole new light, appreciating simple things like being able to breathe, seeing flowers in a neighbor's garden, and receiving a hug or a kind word. Whether you are stressed out, feel discouraged, are looking for a solution to a problem, or want to make changes there is nothing that is not improved in some way with regular walking. Even university studies have shown that there is no health issue that does not benefit from regular walking. Fifteen minutes a day is a good start.

Years back, I remember a gentleman walking by my house several times a day. I don't know how many hours he walked. In the beginning, he was so fat he could not walk straight. His gait was more like a wobble from one side to the other. His face was kind of a bluish red, like in people who are prone to a heart attack, and he breathed heavily. He was wearing earphones, just walking day after day and not paying attention to anything else. Once in a while he pulled out a handkerchief to wipe the sweat off his forehead. I suspected that his doctor must have told him to either walk or he would die.

As time went by, I only saw him two times a day, in the morning and late in the afternoon. I noticed that he had lost weight and that his face was not so red anymore. Then I did not see him at all for months. One morning, I was walking my dog and in front of me was a tall, slender gentleman. He was wearing earphones, steadily walking without looking right or left. I looked and looked. Something seemed familiar about him. And then I remembered: It was his gait, swinging from side to side. Although he was slim now, he still wobbled, and that was how I recognized him. It was hard to believe how this man had changed from heavily overweight with a red face and breathing problems, to a slim, nearly athletic figure with a normal complexion.

Birds fly, animals run, fish swim, and the earth spins. Even trees and grass move in the wind. Life is movement! Walking as little as fifteen minutes every day can make a big difference and get you on the path to youthfulness!

Modern Heroes

There are so many people in our times who managed to turn their lives around, even if we don't hear much about them. They exist just as much today as they did fifty or a hundred years ago. I call them heroes because they struggled against all odds and won the battle.

One of the most dramatic transformations I have witnessed was that of Mr. M., an an ophthalmologist from Arizona. The first time I met him he was quite a sight to behold. He was a tall, fat man with no hair and a swollen red face, forty-three years old at the time. Ugly scars still showed where tumors had been removed from his skull. Dressed in a surgeon's outfit, with his head covered by a green cap, like the ones doctors use when in surgery, he came by bus to see me. Due to his condition, he was no longer able to drive. His unusual outfit for a bus trip had the purpose of protecting him from the sun as well as avoiding curious questions by other passengers.

Medical bills had brought him to the brink of poverty. He could not afford a rental car or an airplane ticket since he had been unable to work. His red, scaly hands were covered with white gloves, and over his head he held an umbrella to shelter himself from the glaring sun. His eyes had become extremely sensitive. He had to wear dark glasses for protection.

As soon as he sat down on a chair in my office he started crying from the tremendous pain in his face and itching hands. He had pain practically all over his body. It must have been so bad that he not only felt it in his body, but in his soul as well. He had been diagnosed with Lupus and some kind of cancer by five doctors, who had all given up on him. His face was swollen. He said that everything was burning and felt so itchy and scaly that he could hardly stand it. While we were talking, he had to keep scratching himself and it nearly broke my heart to see this big, tall man sitting there and cry like a helpless baby. His hair had fallen out, and he showed me the scars on his head and the side of his face where the tumors had been. He felt dizzy, was taking medication for Lupus, anxiety, depression, vertigo, and several other aches and pains. He had bad breath and his hands did not stop trembling. How much worse could he get?

He mentioned he worked Saturdays and Sundays out of necessity, because he had hardly any clients left and was glad when somebody came at all. A few got as far as his store and then escaped with a vague excuse in fear that whatever this man had might be contagious, and they were not eager to catch it.

A simple energy test revealed that he had a fungus and was full of parasites. He started on a cleansing diet. Since none of his medications was for life threatening conditions, like high blood pressure, diabetes, or heart related problems, he decided to drop them all. After a few days, he called to let me know that he had the flu and in some ways felt worse than before. I told him his flu-like symptoms might be a healing crisis and could be considered normal under the circumstances. His body was trying to eliminate all kinds of toxins, including the medications. It would be temporary and afterwards he would start feeling better. I suggested eating more garlic as a natural antibiotic, and, if he was willing, to try enemas. He was willing. He was desperate, and he did whatever it might take to get well, although at that point he had his doubts about the whole process.

A month later he was considerably improved. His hands were still burning, but he had lost sixteen pounds of toxic matter and said that his desire to smoke cigarettes had decreased. He was not taking any of his prescription medications anymore. He said he had been giving himself enemas almost every day. In the beginning, the water was so nasty he had to repeat them an unbelievable six times before it came out clear. He saw live worms coming out. More than anything else, it was probably those disgusting worms coming out of him that convinced him he was on the right track. Once he saw with his own eyes what was coming out of his body with the black, stinking enema water, he realized what had kept him sick, and that drugs were not the answer. He kept cleansing with diet, fasting, and enemas, and as soon as he was able to, he went to the gym for up to two hours every day. He had tried all kinds of medications before and had only gotten worse. Every doctor had told him that there was no cure for him. Inner cleansing was his answer and he was willing to do it.

Over the following months, he experienced several healing crises. At one time, one of his eyes was so swollen he could hardly see. Then his legs felt numb, blood and pus came out of his gums, he had tremendous pain in his ears, could not sleep, his liver ached and he kept vomiting. At times, there was no energy at all and the skin on his face and hands was still dark. But he never lost faith. He never gave up. Every month we changed the program according to his progress and new situation.

He took a workshop on how to heal himself naturally and realized what was causing his condition: toxins, toxins, and more toxins. Gradually, he improved and stopped hiding behind his surgeon's outfit. He began dressing more normal. Soon, both the parasites and the fungus were gone. His skin cleared up. His eyesight improved. The aches and pains disappeared.

He stopped smoking. In little over a year, he lost an astonishing 120 pounds, which were 120 pounds of toxins.

Month after month, there were changes in the way he felt and in his appearance. He looks handsome now, tall and slim, athletic. His energy has come back and he claims he never felt better in his whole life. He still spends about two hours in the gym every day, and the skin on his hands looks soft and tender. I have never seen any man with more beautiful hands! His hair has not grown back due to the scars on his head, but he says he can feel a little fuzz coming. He claims he does not need his eyeglasses anymore either. He is back to normal, better than normal, he would say, because even his business is blooming. For some time now he has been teaching yoga classes on television, and nobody would ever suspect how sick this man had been and how much he had suffered.

Learning from his own experience, he tries to help people holistically. Once a week, he takes a day off and never works on Sundays anymore. He either goes to church thanking God for the miracle he experienced, or just enjoys the day at home. Due to his gentle personality and new-found sense of humor, he has become very popular and made friends with people who share his views on life. When people ask him about the diet that brought him back to life, he just smiles and replies, "God's diet." He fully understands that not everybody is willing to do what it takes or follow in his footsteps, although to him it was worth it. He has become a radiant light to himself and a teacher to others. I feel blessed that our paths have crossed.

Then there is the man they call "The Walking Miracle," a musician from Chicago, who also healed himself naturally after being given up by his doctors. Mr. O. also has an amazing story to tell. This man had not only been given up by the medical establishment, he was just about to give up on himself. In fact, he had already gone to a priest for his last rites and final blessing. For seven years, he had been unable to leave the house, entirely depending on his wife for food, care, and transportation.

Mr. O. had been diagnosed with scleroderma, a deadly disease where the skin hardens and eventually becomes so tight that the affected individual becomes unable to open their mouth and eyes and dies a painful death. When I saw him, his face and hands were terribly swollen and had a blazing red color. Nobody could touch him. Immediately, blood and pus would ooze out of his skin. When his wife drove him to my office, it took him a good ten minutes to get out of the car and slowly walk up to the building, supported by her. Apparently, he was aching all over.

At the time, Mr. O. was close to seventy years of age. There was so much pain in his neck that he was unable to turn his head or look over his shoulders. He tried to make a joke, telling me that he was all *krasno*, which in Russian means red or beautiful, but he could not laugh because the skin around his mouth and eyes was too tight. He said that at night he could not sleep due to the pain in his neck and all over his body. Nothing was easy for him. I remembered him from years back. He was an athlete who participated in many competitions. People thought he was a genius—a genius in music, mathematics, and in languages, speaking at least five of them fluently, among them Russian and Mandarin. It was pitiful to see him now, so small and helpless, confined to this practically useless body and still trying to make jokes and be brave. This man, once so independent, so intelligent, now had to be fed and bathed by his wife.

When he came to see me, he was using cortisone and a number of other drugs the doctors had prescribed over the years. Apparently, they did not help him at all, maybe even made his condition worse. He also suffered from a fungus, which had not been detected previously and which was destroying his body. Mr. O. started on a restricted diet. I don't know how well he followed it, because his wife was too busy to cook for him and there was not much he could do on his own, except faithfully taking the supplements. A month later there was very little improvement. We changed his diet, and again, after another month the improvement was not quite what we had expected. The herbal supplement on its own was not enough and he could not get the fruit and vegetables to follow his diet.

I mentioned urine therapy and suggested he try it. He looked at me as if I had lost my marbles, and just replied, "Why not?" The last thing he wanted to do was offend me or argue since this was his last hope. I could kind of guess his thoughts. He was not convinced at all. Since he was unable to do much of anything and mainly sat at home alone, I suggested he read something about the topic and lent him Martha Christy's wonderful book *Your Own Perfect Medicine* and later on Armstrong's classic on urine therapy, *The Water of Life*. After that, he was convinced and started with a few drops at a time, gradually increasing the daily amount.

Urine therapy is the least expensive treatment. Mr. O. did not have much to lose any more, except for his pride. After a few weeks, he fell into a terrible crisis. It was like a flu with high fever and lasted for days. His wife told him to stop the "foolishness" unless he wanted to die. By now he did not want to give up. He had read those two books about other people's miraculous healing, about their crises, and eventual recovery from ailments about as bad as his own. He continued, hoping for a change for the better. He understood that his body was reacting to the different medications and poisons he had ingested over the years, including cortisone, and was now trying to free itself with fevers and diarrhea. He saw it as the price he had to pay and did not give up. He kept drinking his own urine and followed part of the diet. After the fever subsided, he felt much, much better. There was less pain and for the first time in months, maybe in years, he managed to sleep all night through.

From then on, his progress was very fast. Within weeks, he could walk again on his own. His skin color returned from blazing red to normal, and about four months after his initial visit we went to a restaurant to celebrate his newly found health. He mentioned that none of his friends could believe he was still alive. When he picked up his wife from work, one of her co-workers called him "The walking miracle." Yes, God had done a miracle for him, using a combination of diet and urine therapy. Somebody in his family told me later that not only was he completely normal again, his hair color had gradually turned dark again and that he looked better than his forty-five-year old nephew. Of course, what we eat also determines the composition of our urine.

Another brave person of the outstanding self-healings I remember is a beautiful, young woman, Ms. L, who currently lives in Mexico City. She looks so radiant and full of energy that people doubt it when she tells them that there was a time when she could not walk on her own after being diagnosed with Multiple Sclerosis. This lively, bubbly person was only twenty-five years old when she was diagnosed with the disease. She was swollen, heavily overweight and used a walker to support herself. The sadness in her eyes, and acne on her face and neck made it difficult to fully appreciate her beauty. She had seen just about every specialist in town to consult about her ailments. There was the neurologist, two gastroenterologists, an internist, a urologist, a gynecologist, and a dermatologist.

Between doctor visits she spent time in the hospital for emergency care, all of which had nearly bankrupted her family. She, too, was eager to try anything to recover from her misery. She had already given away her beloved dog, because her support group told her that soon she would no longer be able to care for the dog and that it was in her best interest to leave her husband as well since he would not be willing to carry her or change her diapers as the dreadful disease advanced and she would have no control over her bowel movements.

They asked her to install rails in every room of her house and widen the doors for wheelchair access. Although this lady had been pumped up with steroids, antibiotics, antidepressants and all kinds of prescription drugs, there was no sign of relief. I don't know whether she believed me or not when I told her that the cause for most of her problems might be a fungus.

She changed her diet, started taking herbal supplements, and after a while took daily walks, although they were short in the beginning. To the dismay of her family and support group she stopped all her doctor visits and medication, something she had been told was impossible and would eventually kill her. She decided to join a yoga group and started looking better from month to month. Her weight came down, her skin improved, her hair became glossy again, her eyes took a new sparkle and there was no sign of depression any more.

Since she had been constipated since early childhood, she knew that one of her main problems had to do with her digestion. She tried enemas and sporadically a colonic irrigation in addition to the diet. For some reason, she had a tremendous fear of enemas and believed they would be harmful to her. In my opinion, she needed to be afraid of what stayed inside and not of what was coming out of her. She finally agreed to an enema and told me that she had to flush the toilet five times. What had come out was horrible. Still, she was reluctant to repeat the procedure.

She was willing to improve her diet and go for daily walks. After going through minor healing crises, she now gets a lot of compliments on how healthy she looks. She had a second child, a beautiful boy, and there is no more talk about leaving her husband or installing contraptions for the handicapped in her home. She walks close to an hour several days a week and has traveled on her own to places as far away as New York or California. Nobody who sees her believes it when out of habit she keeps mentioning that she has a terrible disease. She is now confident that she can work again as soon as the baby grows and find a bigger home with a yard for the children.

Each person who has gone the path of self-healing, has changed his or her life afterwards. There is tremendous gratitude just to be alive. It always seems to be the same pattern they followed: a change in diet, inner cleansing, some kind of exercise, like walking outdoors, and most of all, an open mind to search for more natural ways of healing instead of using traditional medicine and never accepting the idea that there is no cure.

Peace After the Storm

Health, wealth and happiness come with a price. We want to look good, feel good, and have plenty of energy. Even if we were born with certain physical privileges, eventually we have to do our part to maintain them. Women use makeup, cosmetic surgery, creams, pills, and ointments to make themselves more attractive. Men too are concerned about their looks but what worries them most is hair loss and their virility. Both, men and women can benefit from improving their diet.

Occasional inner cleansing and exercise help all of us to achieve our goals faster. Cosmetics can make us look better and should not just be used to cover up what we don't like about ourselves. Most problems are due to accumulated toxins. Once we get rid of these toxins our natural beauty will return. Before we feel better, we may temporarily feel terrible, unless we go slowly and improvements also come gradually.

When I initiated my health odyssey, I imagined that by leaving medication and doctors behind I had found an effective, non-invasive alternative and that I would feel good right away. I had no idea how bad one can feel before seeing improvements. When I met Dr. Sperl, I also registered for yoga classes at the same time. The welcome sign at the desk in the yoga studio promised health, wisdom, and self-realization. I did not care much about the latter two. All I wanted was my health back. I attended the classes regularly and was fortunate to study under the guidance of an Indian master. After becoming an initiate, I also practiced meditation, and once a month all disciples met in a group with the Master. He recommended keeping a diary and offered to be of assistance if we needed help.

A few weeks into the yoga classes and following Dr. Sperl's diet at the same time, I got a terrible cold, worse than I had ever had in my whole life. It lasted six weeks. Instead of getting better, it seemed to me that things were getting worse. To say that I was disappointed with the results of my new path is an understatement. I wrote about it in my diary and refused to show it to the Master or talk to him about it. I was not only sick but also mad about the whole situation. I had a fever and everything hurt: my head, my teeth, my spine, my stomach, maybe even my hair. Coughing up phlegm until I was red in the face came with it. I did not take medication as all my well-meaning friends suggested. Once the ordeal was over, to my surprise, I felt great and practically never had another cold again, at least not this bad.

The vegetarian diet, which is highly recommended for yoga students, also did a number on me. With all the salads and vegetarian food, I had painful gas and even vomited a few times. Sometimes I thought the reactions might kill me, but I stuck to the program. To make things worse, I heard about a famous water cure, and without any warning went for it as well. It promised results when everything else failed.

The cure consisted of drinking six times a day, two glasses of distilled water before and after meals. About the third day on the water cure I got unstoppable diarrhea. Nothing I ate stayed inside. It was close to a month before I decided to go and ask my naturopathic doctor what I could do about it. Dr. Sperl shook his head and commented something like I must really have been in a bad state. It nearly seemed as if he was going to congratulate me for my success. He then suggested I eat only grated apples and drink chamomile tea to normalize my digestion. Santo remedio! The diarrhea stopped and I felt good again.

Involuntarily, I had undergone some powerful cleansing processes. It was not until much later that I understood what had happened. It was indeed a good thing, maybe one of the best things that could have happened to me. It was like shaking everything loose inside and making the bad stuff come out. Maybe at the time I was just not ready for such drastic reaction and in my effort to get well soon I probably overdid things. Today, I know that we have the option to go slow and avoid extreme reactions. In those times, I was desperate.

After seeing so many doctors and trying everything without results, I wanted immediate improvements, preferably yesterday. Had I known ahead of time what was in store, I might never have started my adventure into natural healing, but in hindsight I am glad things happened the way they did. The fever, the diarrhea, the cough, the skin eruptions, the pain, everything was my body's effort to get rid of toxic matter. I just had no idea how intoxicated I was.

We all have waste in our body, especially in the colon. For the average person, it is about five pounds. Even people who fast for forty days on water report about nasty stuff still coming out with an enema after twenty, thirty or more days. They also mention a state of well-being afterwards like they never experienced before.

Disease, premature aging, and even death can be caused by toxic matter which is accumulating inside of us. These internal problems then cause a variety of symptoms that show up on the outside. It may be in the form of excess weight, dull hair, skin tags, discolorations, diseased teeth, or brittle nails; it can be through aches and pains, sexual problems, infertility, insomnia, shortness of breath, and high blood pressure. Cleansing is a simple, inexpensive way to reverse all these symptoms and return to health. Simple practices, like drinking a glass of water with lemon juice in the morning, eating more salads and a daily walk may prevent us from ever having to deal with major health issues.

When toxins leave the body, it can happen in the form of a flu, through diarrhea, skin outbreaks, puss, vomiting, swellings or a fever. The body will try in every possible way to eliminate them. The process is unpleasant, but the results are worth it. Some people get headaches or experience nausea. Sometimes toxins and fluids are moved from vital organs towards the extremities where they are less dangerous. We might then wonder why our hands or ankles are swollen. Seeing stuff coming to the surface can be scary.

Inner cleansing is like a house cleaning. We are mostly unaware of all the dirt and rust, and cobwebs that have accumulated over time until we do a thorough cleaning. When we wash the curtains, clean the rugs, remove dirt from under the sink, and wipe kitchen and bathroom cabinets clean, it feels like the energy in the whole house changed. It is kind of lighter. The same with our body. We feel alive again, rejuvenated, and more energized after removing those toxins. Sometimes even the neighbors look friendlier afterwards.

The sicker a person is, the more reactions there will be. Somebody in good shape will hardly experience any discomfort at all. Remembering my own experience, I always suggest people go slow. It is important to first understand what is happening.

When you initiate a cleansing process through diet, fasting, or enemas you may see some nauseating stuff going down the toilet. With it goes disease. The body releases mucus, slime, fungus, and substances that should not be there. Some people see worms coming out. Strange smells and colors might indicate the presence of heavy metals. Afterwards, your skin will be clearer, your eyes brighter, your energy increased, and your thinking will be a little sharper. Friends might wonder whether you lost weight, changed your hairstyle, or whether it is a new kind of makeup you are wearing. You will look more radiant and they can't pinpoint what exactly is different about you. You just look so much better, often in a matter of weeks. Subtle changes take place after an inner cleansing. In hindsight, we come to understand that these crises are a blessing.

Yogis know a lot about health. Their Holy Scriptures, the Vedas, include many details on diet and other practices which have been around for thousands of years. Some teachers are over a hundred years old and never look older than in their thirties. They consider their bodies to be God's temple and take good care of it. It is not vanity. They like to enjoy a long life with the goal to serve humanity. Some yogis share their secrets with their disciples and it is at the discretion of the student whether to follow the advice or not. One of the most valuable purification processes I learned from Swami was the week of discipline, usually carried out during Christmas and the New Year. It is a way to start the New Year in excellent spirits.

The program recommended by Swami includes physical and spiritual practices. During the entire week between Christmas and the New Year he recommends eating only one meal a day, preferably vegetarian. If you are hungry, fruit is allowed for the rest of the day. He also recommended practicing yoga postures. You can walk for an hour or less outdoors instead. Swami encouraged all disciples to read the scriptures and meditate an hour every day.

Each time I practiced these disciplines, I started the New Year feeling better than ever. As I am getting busier, I have reduced the time dedicated to reading the scriptures and meditating, but I still try and limit myself to one meal a day and walk outdoors every day during the entire week.

I believe that these suggestions are helpful for anybody who wishes to improve their health. On one occasion, I shared them with a cheerful young seminary student. To my surprise, he said, "We do this all the time." In other words, eating in moderation, exercising, praying or meditating and reading the scriptures can keep us balanced in everyday life. What a beautiful way to live!

The Power of Vibration

There are many ways our body talks to us, mainly through wellbeing or pain. Even if we try everything possible to achieve wellness, sometimes we get off the path and have to suffer the consequences. In either case, it is amazing how fast our body responds, sometimes within days.

Morgan Spurlock, producer of the documentary *Supersize Me* wanted to prove things for himself. He lived on a healthy diet, but was curious as to what would happen if he did otherwise. He subjected himself to an experiment, which was supervised by three medical doctors. Starting out healthy, he decided that for thirty days all he would eat was food from McDonald's. In the beginning, he had good energy and weighed 185 pounds. at 6'2". His blood pressure was ideal at 120/80 and so was his cholesterol level.

On the second day of the diet, his body reacted with nausea and vomiting, occasional sweating, and twitching in his arms. After five days, he felt too weak to exercise and had already gained some extra weight. Around the twentieth day on the new diet his vital signs had deteriorated to such a degree that all three doctors advised him to discontinue the experiment. By now, his heartbeat had become irregular and he had a fatty liver. He experienced weakness and breathing problems. Nevertheless, he continued.

At the end of thirty days he had gained twenty-five pounds, his blood pressure went up to 140/90, and his cholesterol measured 225, an increase of fifty-six points! He felt depressed and reported that his sex life was almost nonexistent by now. Fortunately, when the experiment was over and he returned to his former healthy lifestyle, he was able to reverse all damages within two months.

In recent years, it has been discovered that we do not depend on the chemical nature of nutrients alone. Our well-being depends to a great deal on the electro-magnetic energy in our body. The higher the frequency, the healthier we are, and this frequency can be influenced by the food we eat and the thoughts we think.

Everything in the Universe is energy, without exception. In order to create the best possible state of health we might want to learn how we can use this knowledge to our advantage. A French electrician by the name of André Simoneton came up with a device called a vitalimeter, which serves to measure the energy frequencies in the human body. He found out that food has its own vibration, and established a relationship between the two. In 1971, he published his findings in a book entitled *Radiations des Aliments, Ondes Humaine et Santé (Vibrations of Food, inside the Human Body, and Health).* He concluded that when a person is alive, his or her electromagnetic frequencies are in a range between 6,200 and 7,100 Angstrom. However, being alive is not the same as being healthy. When our energy drops below 6,500 Å, disease shows up.

Mr. Simoneton's findings are extremely important since they indicate how our state of health continuously varies in accordance with the frequencies present, and these frequencies can be changed by what we put into our body. If we maintain a high frequency, or at least keep it above 6,500 Å, we are likely to enjoy excellent health. Only when we allow our energy to drop can illness appear.

In the Western world, we tend to focus on symptoms, but have no idea where or how they originate. For instance, when we experience an eye problem, we go to an eye doctor and ask him for help. For kidney stones, we would see a different specialist, and so on and so forth. We would treat the symptoms. Another way of looking at health and disease is that the body itself produces these symptoms and it is also the one that does the healing. Now, the question is why do different people suffer from different diseases? When there is a lack of health, the weakest area of the body will start failing first, which varies with each person. It will then affect other areas because everything is related. There is only health or the lack of it, and the only difference between the two is the number of symptoms or the difference in vibration.

As an example, we can take bad teeth. Poor oral health is a sign of poor health in general, and drilling and crowning individual bad teeth does not stop the problem. Only a change in the internal environment can detain the damage. The same applies to everything else. Glasses do not strengthen our optic nerve and insulin shots lower blood sugar as long as their effect lasts. Both control the problem, but do not do much in the way of healing. The body heals itself by raising its vibration, which in turn may happen through our food choices.

Mr. Simoneton's findings do not concern themselves with particular problems. All he is saying is that when our energy drops, any number of symptoms may appear and when we manage to raise the frequency of our vibrations, good health is likely to return. Symptoms tend to appear in the weakest area first, which is the reason why different people have different ailments. For instance, if somebody eats spoiled food (low energy), one person may start vomiting, another person may get headaches. Somebody else may feel tired or get diarrhea. Any kind of intoxication, whether through food or drugs, drastically lowers our vibrations. When these frequencies drop, symptoms appear. When the energy goes up, the body heals and the symptoms disappear.

As long as our frequencies remain above 6,500 Å, bacteria, germs, and viruses do not have much power over us because their energy is lower. They do not find an appropriate terrain to propagate and our immune system remains strong.

Another example is the flu. It is contagious, but not everybody gets it. The answer is inside. When our immune system is weak and our energetic frequency is low, we may catch a disease. However, when we keep our energy level up, no serious disease can touch us. There is no need for shots or expensive medications. It simply cannot happen.

Mr. Simoneton's chart in relation to food is divided into four groups:

1) **Superior Foods** are of high nutritional value (in a range between 6,500 and 10,000 Å). They include fresh fruits and their juices, grains and products from organically grown whole grain, nuts, seeds and their oils, raw and some steamed vegetables, as well as a few animal products like smoked ham, fresh raw fish, shellfish, freshly churned butter, cream, unfermented cheese, and eggs gathered the same day. These are foods that help us maintain excellent health.

2) **Supporting foods** (3,000 to 6,500 Å) maintain our present state of health. Here we find raw milk, regular butter, eggs, honey, raw sugar, wine, vegetables cooked in water, as well as cooked fish. Foods in this group are not powerful enough to produce permanent wellbeing, neither do they harm us.

3) **Inferior foods** are those that promote premature aging, fatigue, and chronic disease. Their frequency lies below 3,000 Å. We want to avoid them as much as possible. They are cooked meat, viscera, sausages, eggs more

than two weeks old, pasteurized milk, coffee, black tea, chocolate, marmalade, fermented cheeses and white bread.

It is interesting to observe that the average Western diet consists of foods from the third category, which infallibly leads to disease. Things get worse when we add items from the fourth category:

Dead foods. They have no measurable vibration and are generally detrimental to our health, like canned food, margarine, alcohol, liquor, refined sugar, baby food, and pastries.

Since the food we consume nourishes our cells, builds our blood, and then forms tissues and organs, the choices we make are decisive for our overall well-being. Nutrition goes far beyond calories, vitamins, minerals, fats, and protein. It mainly depends on its electromagnetic energy. Dead, processed foods with little energy or minerals in them cannot sustain an exuberant state of health. When we improve our diet, the results may be increased energy, prolonged youthfulness, a healthy body in its normal weight, clear skin, improved eyesight, sound sleep at night, good digestion, and love for life in general. Men often are interested in an improved sex life. Sex is part of overall health and will rise or fall with their general state of health. Raising our vibration may improve our sex life and in women fertility.

It is amazing how diet can either make us sick or bring us back to health. Over the years, I have witnessed the process many, many times. Everything we ingest influences our wellbeing. Foods with a higher frequency always produce a superior state of physical, mental, and emotional health. My observation is that the foods mentioned in the higher categories coincide with a higher degree of alkalinity.

Dr. Simoneton does not comment anything on fasting or on the use of drugs, prescribed or others. I would put fasting in the highest category, since we practically live on pure energy when we do not eat at all. Drugs of a chemical nature, whether prescribed or bought over the counter, as well as the use of X-rays and chemotherapy, in my observation, fall into a category of negative vibrations. They are foreign to our body and, therefore, cannot produce health. Of course, in some cases they are lifesaving, especially in an emergency, but in the long run no drug is health building. Drugs should be reduced as soon as possible and substituted with a healthier way of life.

Food Pyramid:

FOOD FRECUENCY AND HUMAN HEALTH

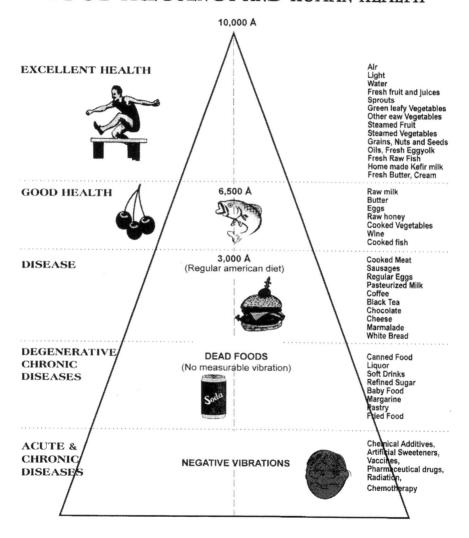

10,000 A

EXCELLENT HEALTH

Air
Light
Water
Fresh fruit and juices
Sprouts
Green leafy Vegetables
Other eaw Vegetables
Steamed Fruit
Steamed Vegetables
Grains, Nuts and Seeds
Oils, Fresh Eggyolk
Fresh Raw Fish
Home made Kefir milk
Fresh Butter, Cream

GOOD HEALTH

6,500 A

Raw milk
Butter
Eggs
Raw honey
Cooked Vegetables
Wine
Cooked fish

DISEASE

3,000 A
(Regular american diet)

Cooked Meat
Sausages
Regular Eggs
Pasteurized Milk
Coffee
Black Tea
Chocolate
Cheese
Marmalade
White Bread

DEGENERATIVE CHRONIC DISEASES

DEAD FOODS
(No measurable vibration)

Canned Food
Liquor
Soft Drinks
Refined Sugar
Baby Food
Margarine
Pastry
Fried Food

ACUTE & CHRONIC DISEASES

NEGATIVE VIBRATIONS

Chemical Additives,
Artificial Sweeteners,
Vaccines,
Pharmaceutical drugs,
Radiation,
Chemotherapy

An Amazing Woman

Any cleansing program or a diet with fruit and vegetables increases our vibration. Talking about "frequency" and "vibration" may sound a little technical, but it is a fact that once we reach higher levels our health, energy and looks will improve. At that time advancements in other areas will occur as well.

One of my clients by the name of Amber is a good example. She was overweight and never had the willpower to do something about it. Sometimes she started a diet and then soon gave up because either she did not see results or because she had no need for it. Her husband took care of everything, and her children loved her the way she was. Of course, she would have liked to improve her looks but the effort was not worth it to her. Following a diet and changing our lifestyle requires some discipline, which she did not have. She was not motivated. Why travel 100 miles an hour and get nauseated when you can enjoy the landscape at twenty miles an hour? She was in a comfortable place just the way she was.

I had known Amber for some time. Her husband brought her in for weight loss once in a while but we never saw much difference. After having given birth to three children and dedicating most of her time to her family she did not care about anything else. She was short and heavy, with a blotchy complexion, no energy, and living mainly on junk food with lots of candy, which ruined her teeth. She looked as if she did not take care of herself, hiding herself and her low self-esteem in old baggy pants.

Her husband was twenty years older than Amber and together they had three children, two of them adults from a previous marriage. He worked as a carpenter, taking care of the family. Amber did not drive and could not speak English. She depended on her husband for everything from food and money to driving her around to wherever she needed to go. Her husband took the children to school, did the shopping, took his wife to doctors' appointments and provided whatever they needed. Amber would totally depend on him. Then one day, completely unexpected, he died of a heart attack. His family tried to take the house from her, and with no financial support and no skills she was wondering how to survive. She fought back and managed at least to stay with her children in the house her husband had left. By necessity she learned to drive a car and for very little money bought an old clunker. She then attended self-improvement classes and learnt to speak English. Her children helped with odd jobs, so they had some money coming in. For her own sake and that of the children, she then decided to take better care of herself and lose some weight.

Time went by and I did not see her again until about two years later. I could not believe my eyes. This woman, who had been living in her husband's shadow, never able to accomplish anything on her own, was a different woman now. She had lost over thirty pounds, had a beautiful complexion, and instead of the baggy pants she used to wear she now wore a sexy black dress. She looked very attractive, maybe even younger than before. Her eyes were sparkling. She had her teeth fixed and now had a pretty smile. Her transformation was so impressive that I asked her what she had been doing. She was proud of what she had accomplished and happy to share her story.

Confronted with her husband's sudden death, Amber at first entered into a state of shock. She then realized that she had to go on, at least for the sake of the children. She was aware of the fact that she did not have much of an education and that she needed to at least change something in her life to have success. No matter how many wonderful inner qualities a person may have, people go by what they see, whether it is in a relationship, in a job environment or in social circles. Her priority was to at least shed some of those extra pounds. Plastic surgery and liposuction were out of the question due to her lack of money. She knew a little bit about diets but prior to this point she never felt an urge to follow any of them. Her husband took care of everything, and that was all she needed. Now her situation had changed. Feeling better and looking presentable had become a matter of survival. The least costly plan for her was to go on a fruit diet, and that is what she did.

For an entire month, Amber lived exclusively on fruit, alternating with freshly squeezed lemon juice and plenty of water. She had also heard about the miracles of urine therapy and decided to give it a try and add it as a secret ingredient. Within a month she lost more than thirty pounds. Her energy and self-discipline increased. Her self-esteem grew. People started complimenting her on her beautiful complexion and she felt encouraged to dress better and sell beauty products.

Soon she bought a better car and started taking English lessons, both of which helped to increase the business. She also took more self-improvement classes. I asked her how she got her clients without speaking English and she said that when people asked her in the workshops what she was doing, she told them about the beauty products she was selling and gave them her card.

It is quite a challenge to live on fruit for a whole month. Amber did it with astounding results. Not only did she experience a physical transformation, her whole life changed. After a year, she met a man her own age. They fell in love and have a beautiful baby girl. Her transformation started with her diet. Maybe she was desperate and had no other choices. She followed through and lived on nothing but fruit for an entire month. She now is an inspiration to others. She also proved that once you start feeling better about yourself, other things start changing as well. I admire her immensely. She started with nothing: no money, no car, very little education and nobody to support her. Once she got started, the results were spectacular. Amber has stayed young well beyond her years, ready to cope with life's challenges.

Trust God and Your Own Judgment!

Everything happens for a reason. Whatever happens in our life, happens with our participation, even if it is not with the desired outcome. If we want different results we need to make better choices. It is easy to blame somebody else but as long as we believe that whatever happens to us is another's fault, we become the victim. Worse, not only go things bad, we attract more negativity in other areas of our life as well. It could be in the area of health, employment, finances, or relationships. It does not matter whether we understand the laws of cause and effect or not, either way we have to deal with the consequences.

For a positive outcome, we need to take positive action. It is that simple. Sometimes we trust others, believing they know better or have more experience, because they mean well, are professionals, or because they say they are psychic. The truth is, nobody knows our situation better than we do and it is okay to make mistakes. We can learn from them and hopefully do better next time.

Some of the people we tend to trust blindly are medical doctors. Whatever they say, we accept their word for it. After all, they have studied and know what is going on inside of us. Do they really? Or are they human beings and there is a possibility they make mistakes too? Usually they base their evaluation on clinical experience. Other times we may wonder how they arrive at their conclusions. One such case was that of a well known local accountant. He was in his sixties and worked for a big company. He hardly ever got sick but one day he got dizzy and had to lie down. He was worried and went to see his doctor. After a thorough examination, the doctor told him he could not find anything wrong with him and that the dizziness was probably because the man was so tall. I wondered about that because the man had been tall all his life. Besides, not all tall people get dizzy.

Another story is that of my father. One day in October he came home and had to lie down. He was so depressed because the doctor told him that he would not be around for Christmas. Christmas came and went and nothing happened. Then there was Easter and another year went by. My father still lived another sixteen years, and the physician died years before him.

I also remember a wonderful neighbor of mine, Mr. Vance. His hands were deformed from arthritis. I asked him whether he was taking anything for his arthritis. He said he didn't and that he was disappointed with the medical profession. Last time he saw a doctor, he was prescribed Prozac for his condition. He wondered why, because he was not suffering from depression nor was he suicidal. All he wanted was to get rid of his pain. The doctor told him that he recommended Prozac because it was all in his head. Being in terrible pain and deformed, all in his mind? I wonder in what medical school they teach that severe arthritis is a mental problem.

Nowadays, more and more people are being put on medication being told that they are "pre" something or the other. If you are pre-diabetic or pre-cancerous, it means that you don't have the problem. Of course, you may get it, like everybody else. We all may, and it sounds reasonable to take medication in a preemptive way, except for the fact that all medication has side effects and people often start getting precisely the disease they want to prevent.

Before you do what others say, always check it out first. Get more information or a second opinion. Nobody is perfect and we can all make mistakes, even trained professionals. If you are not sure what to do, ask questions, particularly about risks and side effects. We need our medical professionals and their expertise, but the truth is they are human and can err. Sometimes these mistakes can be costly and irreversible.

For the majority of people, it is hard to understand that the body has a natural tendency to heal itself. All a medical doctor can do is state the facts, give a name to the problem and write a prescription. Some people love to talk about their ailments and pride themselves on the amount of medication they are taking. Their symptoms may be controlled, but there will be no real long-term improvement.

We would be better off if we accepted that we created our problems; and if we are the ones who created them, we are also the ones who can create something different. Almost all symptoms can be reversed. We play an important role in our own healing process and sometimes miracles happen. My father was such a case and although he did not change anything in his lifestyle, he still lived for many years. Maybe he simply accepted the fact that death is inevitable and began to appreciate the little things of everyday life.

In any case, before trusting anybody blindly, it is always good to become more knowledgeable, to educate ourselves. Reading about disease is a way to convince ourselves that we have all the symptoms. Doctors study disease, not health, and they believe that everybody has some ailment. One doctor declared openly that there are no healthy persons, only those who have not been examined enough. Your doctor will not tell you that you might get well without his help or that the disease might disappear on its own. He will not suggest the exclusive use of herbs, exercise, or a change in diet, first of all, because he does not believe in them. Most doctors do not believe in the body's capability to regenerate itself.

Whether you go the natural way or opt for surgery, always use common sense and, if possible, try natural things without side effects first. A friend from Switzerland told me about her uncle who was ready to have surgery. A well-meaning relative gave him a book on raw food. The more he read, the more interested he became. Immediately, he started eating everything raw, even potatoes. He took a risk and never had the surgery.

Once people hear the word "incurable" they get fearful. They think that they have to act fast, trusting that traditional treatments are the only way out, even if statistics prove the opposite. For a few, a negative diagnosis may become a wake-up call and they start looking for alternatives. There is no guarantee of recovery either way, but more people have attained superior health with a healthy lifestyle than with drugs, chemotherapy, and radiation. Natural therapies have been around for thousands of years. The Indian Master Osho mentions in one of his books that as far back as 5,000 years ago people in India had such advanced techniques for surgery as we do today, even brain surgery. They gave everything up in favor of Ayurveda, the science of life, with the goal to achieve a better quality of life afterwards.

Sometimes we don't get immediately what we ask for and other things improve first. Nature always knows what to do and in the right sequence. One of my clients came in to lose weight. After a month she called me, a little disappointed, because she had not lost any weight at all, but she admitted that her hair did not fall out anymore and that her period had become more normal.

There is a story about a woman who wanted to get pregnant. She prayed to God for a son. God agreed. When her time came, she gave birth to a beautiful baby girl. She reminded God of His promise and asked if He had made a mistake. God told her again that she would have a boy. The next child was another girl. Surely, God would not lie to her and He had promised a boy. So, she had another talk with Him. He assured her that she would have a boy. The third child was a boy. She was overjoyed and thanked God for her newborn son. God asked her about the two girls. She said she adored them. They were such wonderful children. God smiled and replied that if He had given her the boy right in the beginning, she would not have had her two daughters. He then asked her if she would have preferred it that way. The woman now understood that everything is for a reason and comes to us when the timing is right.

Diet for Beauty

When I look in the mirror, I see quite a bit of imperfection. Where is the smooth complexion, the shiny hair, the slim body, the attractive smile of younger years? Life leaves its traces. Sometimes we gain weight and feel overweight. Sometimes we feel underweight. Our energy is not the same any more either. Hair gets thinner. Wrinkles show up. I know I have changed. I may never be perfect, but at least I can do something to stay healthy and slow down the aging process.

At some point we are willing to pay high prices for beauty treatments, and in some cases even for plastic surgery. Aging is a process, which we can slow down and sometimes reverse. I often hear people say that all they want is to be healthy. We can strive for more. Often, they are surprised when after a month of changing their diet they have lost weight, their energy has improved, their hair is more manageable, and certain skin problems have disappeared. They look younger and feel better. Good health shows up as beauty. Age does not exclude beauty. Beyond the physical, there are other attractive traits like education, a cheerful attitude, being open-minded, and orderly. It is doable, although in everyday life our physical appearance is quite important.

My lifelong dream has been to have a clear, rosy complexion. I think I was born with freckles. My mother had freckles. My father had freckles. And I had them. My freckles bothered me, and later my age spots bothered me some more. I tried everything possible to get rid of them. When I was about twelve years old somebody told me that frogs' eggs would bleach the skin. After school I went to a nearby pond and put a handful of those frogs' eggs on my face. Apparently, they had to be left on to dry. I just hoped nobody would see me on my way home. The freckles never went away. I then tried different creams and potions. Some irritated my skin. Others made the problem worse after I stopped using them. The only thing that helped a bit was a change in diet and inner cleansing. My forehead, where I used no creams at all, had the nicest skin.

I also noticed improvements after participating in a seven-day juice fast in Arizona. Most of the participants used to live on raw food only. How beautiful they looked! Regardless of their age and sex, they all looked radiant and had the prettiest complexions, men and women alike. Some alternated fasting and cleanses with raw food, others were not 100 percent on a raw food diet and occasionally included brown rice or vegetables.

As far as I know, they all followed vegan diets, meaning they ate no animal products whatsoever, like honey, eggs, or cheese. Even the babies, who were raised on mother's milk and raw food from birth, impressed me with their bright clear eyes and cheerful little personalities. There were people in their thirties, forties, and even seventies from different continents and ethnic backgrounds. They all looked fit and happy. Enjoying the hot pools of natural spring water, it seemed that nobody had a care in the world. It truly felt like paradise. The place is known as Eden Hot Springs.

I am still grateful to David Wolfe, who organized the retreat. He is a leader in juicing and raw foods and also the author of several books. So many of us benefited from the week of fresh juices, enlightening talks, the pools, the sunshine, and each other's company. David is one of the most knowledgeable, yet simplest, most joyful, and charismatic people I have ever met. I cannot say enough about how energetic, compassionate, honest, patient and truly beautiful he is. He has a genuine passion for whatever he is doing and a great sense of humor, sometimes bordering on the hilarious when he answers questions. He talks the talk, and also walks the walk.

Focusing on our problems does not get us far. Instead, we can visualize how we want to be and learn from others, moving in the direction of our goals. Whether we actually get to experience all the health, wealth, and happiness we desire remains open. The path to get there is important. Whether we are overweight, suffer from cellulite, arthritis, insomnia, skin tags, hair falling out, poor eyesight, varicose veins, premature wrinkles or low energy, most of these symptoms can be reversed, sometimes completely, others to a certain degree. Worrying does not help, action does, and it may imply sacrifices. Maybe we have to give up candies, do more exercise, eat fewer meals a day or support the body in its cleansing actions.

Animals retain their natural beauty throughout life. We can learn from them, especially regarding food and movement. Animals never eat three meals a day. Some of them do not even get to eat once every day. In times of scarcity and sickness, they do not eat at all. During hibernation, some of them live without food for months and nothing bad happens to them. Wild animals eat everything raw, sticking to one kind of food only, like grasses, grains, or meat. They only drink water. Movement, alternating with times of rest, is very important. Birds and insects fly, fish swim, and land animals run, walk or crawl. In other words: they live in accordance with the laws of nature.

Whatever we do, even to live a simple life, requires discipline to see results. The famous financial adviser Suze Orman said, "You can either have success or you can make excuses, but you cannot have both." She is right. We have to take action. The results are then our reward and encouragement to go a step further. Sometimes it takes more time than anticipated to get results. Instead of going from miserable to great, we might have to experience something worse before we get better. Don't give up! Difficulties are not the end. They can be the beginning of something much better coming along.

When I was a child, my father taught me a valuable lesson. He used to carry me on his shoulders and, no matter what he said or did, he was my hero. One day I fell and scratched my knee. Immediately, I started crying. My father tried to convince me that I could go on despite the impact. With a smile on his face he said, "You are a brave girl. Show me that it does not hurt. Throw yourself down again!" I had my doubts because it hurt quite a bit. But then my father was never wrong. Hesitantly, I threw myself on the ground a second time, careful not to fall on the same knee. It distracted me and I stopped crying, although I was not convinced that this was as much fun as my father seemed to believe.

Later on, when I happened to fall again, without my father being present, I threw myself down a second time, showing the world that such a little mishap did not bother me at all and that indeed I was a brave girl and did not cry. As I grew older, I started feeling silly throwing myself down a second time. Nobody else did that! But I was still in the habit. I first looked around to make sure nobody was looking. Eventually, I learned that falling one time was embarrassing enough. There was no need for repetition. I would just get up and move on.

Maybe this was one of the most valuable lessons I ever learned. There will always be obstacles. However, we can overcome them and life goes on. It is our choice to dwell on lack, pain and separation or move towards the good things that are on their way.

Sometimes fasting and changing our diet is not enough. Nowadays our soils are so depleted that we may have to take supplements. Probiotics boost our immune system. They increase our good intestinal flora, where 80 percent of the immune system is located. Purified ocean water contains over a hundred minerals and trace minerals. In some areas, ocean water is used to obtain better crops. Then there are sea vegetables and greens like Spirulina, chlorella, alfalfa or raw spinach, all full of nutrients. Fresh garlic is another miracle food to boost the immune system. It is a natural antibiotic without negative side effects. A raw egg yolk can be added to a smoothie or mixed in a glass of freshly squeezed orange juice. It contains everything the human body needs, except for vitamin C. Skin and hair will benefit tremendously when we take it over a certain period of time.

Cod liver oil maintains skin and bone health, and with its high amount of Vitamin A it may improve our eyesight as well. Enzymes, although already contained in raw foods, benefit our digestive system and keep us young beyond our years.

A newly popularized star among supplements due to its extraordinary benefits for health and beauty is **bone broth**. Being vegetarian, I have a little resistance to drinking it. Bone broth is sold in powder form in health food stores and one can mix a scoopful in hot water and drink it once or twice a day. Bone broth is full of important minerals. It also has some protein and dietary fiber. It contains collagen, glucosamine, chondroitin, and hyaluronic acid to support the digestive system and improve joint health. It also keeps our skin supple and is believed to strengthen hair and fingernails. It supports liver function, and is excellent for cleansing and detoxification of the body. Bone broth alkalizes the body (very important!) and prevents loss of muscle. Drinking the broth keeps you from feeling hungry.

People who consume it say it helps them lose weight, sleep more soundly at night, and have more energy during the day. In other words, it seems to be an absolute miracle for rejuvenation. I was in doubt whether to buy a can or not, when the sales clerk told me that one of our local beauty queens buys it regularly. She also mentioned that one of her co-workers at the store takes the product and has seen dramatic changes in the beauty of her skin. In powder form, it is practically tasteless and odorless. All one needs to do is add a cup of warm water to a tablespoon or two of the powder. With vitamin C it is supposed to be more effective.

Another supplement for health and beauty worth mentioning is MSM (Methylsulfonylmethane). Its name sounds chemical, but MSM is nothing but organic sulfur, which naturally occurs in fruit, vegetables, and rain water. Sulfur is called the beauty mineral because it improves hair growth, keeps our skin smooth, and strengthens our nails. It keeps our joints flexible and detoxifies the liver. Sulfur is involved in more than 150 functions, benefiting enzyme production, our hormones, antibody formation, and acts as a free radical scavenger. MSM has a bitter taste, especially if the body is low in it. Whether you take it in capsule form or as a powder diluted with water, it is more effective in combination with vitamin C or lemon juice, which can also mask the taste and speed up the formation of collagen.

These and other supplements used with consistency bring noticeable improvements. They may also be added to a smoothie like the one a client of mine came up with. She mixes:

1/2 an apple
a pear or some slices of papaya
2 tablespoons of oats
2 tablespoons of ground flaxseeds
a handful of spinach
1 teaspoon of blue-green algae, Spirulina or chlorella,
and enough water to fill the blender

It makes about three glasses and can give you a good start for the day, replacing cooked food. If you don't have to kiss any co-workers, you may want to add a clove of garlic to the brew, and Chia seeds for extra energy. One can live on this smoothie forever without the need for other food. When you start the day with this power drink, health and beauty will increase, regardless of what happens later on in the day. It is hard to believe that something so rejuvenating can taste so delicious as well.

European Spa Diet

O f all the rejuvenation diets, this is one of my favorites because it is easy to follow and does not make you hungry. This famous diet, named after the Austrian physician Franz Xaver Mayr (1875-1965), has become popular in modern European spas due to its simplicity and long-lasting rejuvenating effects. Although it is considered a fasting and cleansing diet, during the entire time you are on it, you will hardly ever feel hungry, especially if on the new version, which allows the addition of other foods after the first week.

Dr. Mayr grew up in Austria, where as a boy he helped his father take care of the sheep and cows on the family farm. He later studied medicine and while working as a medical doctor in a well-known health center he noticed that almost all the patients suffered from digestive problems and constipation. Regardless of the nature of their ailments, they all seemed to be related to the digestive system, causing changes in their complexion, their facial expression, and body shape. When Dr. Mayr put them on a gentle diet of rolls and raw milk, not only did their digestion improve, but to everybody's amazement the program had dramatic effects on other seemingly unrelated organs like the heart, liver, kidneys and the reproductive system as well.

His main idea was to soothe the intestine, to cleanse it, and then retrain it towards normal functioning. Dr. Mayr achieved all three of them with a simple diet of rolls and raw milk, with an emphasis on conscious chewing. According to his observations, improper eating habits caused distention of the small intestine, where fermentation and putrefaction tend to generate poisons. Once they are absorbed into the blood stream, they affect all cells and organs of the body, causing a variety of symptoms. When the good intestinal flora has been disturbed, disease-causing bacteria multiply readily. This in turn affects the immune system and we become more prone to disease. When toxic matter is no longer eliminated sufficiently, other organs have to take over. They then start breaking down due to an overload followed by acute and chronic diseases. Even mental and emotional problems like depression, irritability, or memory loss can all be attributed to problems in the intestinal tract. Likewise, when the intestinal flora is restored and digestion improves, a person's whole outlook on life starts changing as well.

Dr. Mayr recommended twenty-one days for the cure or longer. During this time, the patient eats only one or two semi-dry rolls a day together with a few sips of raw whole milk. The key to success is the **chewing**. Dr. Mayr recommended that each bite be chewed at least thirty times, possibly longer, until it gets completely liquefied in the mouth. Most of us do not chew our food long enough, and thereby do not allow the body to produce sufficient digestive enzymes.

Why white bread? White bread offers practically no nutrition at all. It gives the intestine a rest. And that is the key! The rolls just serve to practice our chewing and to release valuable digestive enzymes. To eat one roll like this might take a good part of the morning, probably training one's patience as well. The raw whole milk, on the other hand, provides such complete nutrition that one can live on it exclusively for a very long time. It is easy to digest and rich in vitamins, minerals, proteins, fat, and natural enzymes, all in the right proportion. It allows the intestinal flora to renew itself.

In a clinical environment, the program is supervised by a physician specially trained in the Mayr therapy. He examines the patient in the beginning of the cure and daily administers a suggested abdominal massage to activate peristalsis. He also observes the progress of each patient and sometimes recommends special herbal teas in accordance with their needs as well as breathing exercises and daily warm abdominal wraps. It is all about cleansing and a return to normal bowel function. The cure is so simple that most people can follow it at home without risk. At home, it is less costly and therefore can be followed for a longer period of time. There is no need to take time off from work. Most people feel good all the time.

Although the entire process is mostly about learning to chew properly, there are a few more things to know. The goal is to soothe, cleanse, and gradually regenerate the intestinal tract. Cleansing starts in the morning with a purifying drink. During the entire duration of the cure, one starts the day with a glass of water in which one heaped teaspoon of Epsom salts (magnesium sulfate) has been dissolved. In Europe, they call the Epsom salts bitter salts. This bitter water rinses the intestine, flushing out toxic matter embedded in the intestinal walls. It also allows poisons that have been loosened up from other areas to pour into the intestine. Usually a good bowel movement follows about half an hour after taking the bitter water. It is normal for the stools to be liquid or very loose.

For the first two weeks, or even longer, the bowel movements might be dark and smelly. Also, the urine may turn out to be more concentrated than usual or you may recognize a strange smell coming off your skin. The entire body is undergoing a detoxification process and it is highly recommended to drink at least two to three quarts of water or herbal teas during the day to activate elimination. One may follow the program for any length of time. Ideally, it is recommended to last between twenty-one and forty days to reverse longstanding problems.

Then, at least half an hour after the water with the Epsom salts, one may start with breakfast, consisting of a hard roll and some milk. Each bite is to be chewed at least thirty times until it liquefies in your mouth and then you take a sip of the milk. This makes for better absorption of the nutrients in the milk. Since it is hard to get day-old white bread in the United States, I prefer to cut my roll or bread into slices and then toast each side lightly. This gives it a very pleasant taste.

The second "meal" of the day is exactly the same, only now you call it lunch. To give the intestine a better rest these two are the only solid meals, unless you are very hungry and then another roll is permitted in the evening. In the afternoon, you only sip herbal teas, if desired, sweetened with raw honey. The cure should be pleasant, with the goal towards improved elimination, as well as resting and rebuilding of the good intestinal flora. Healthy weight loss and overall improved metabolic functions will be the result. If you have the time and money, you can go to a spa and get the supervision of a trained physician. The results from weight loss to overall rejuvenation are reported to be outstanding, particularly as far as skin and energy are concerned.

In the U.S., it might not be easy to obtain raw milk. For human consumption, its sale is limited. Pasteurized, homogenized, deodorized milk with growth hormones and antibiotics that were given to the cows is not the same. What once used to be a whole food has been made completely useless, if not harmful. The effects of altering the milk are so severe that even a calf will die within weeks of drinking pasteurized milk. It is interesting to know that the Food and Drug Administration, who controls the sale of raw milk, only allows it for pets, and states that feeding cats and dogs with pasteurized milk can be life threatening to them. If pasteurized milk can kill a cat, a dog, or a calf, how good can it be for humans?

Anyway, if the sale of raw milk to the public is not permitted in your state, maybe there is an opportunity to become part of a cow-share program. Such shares are not costly and make the consumption of raw milk legal. As an alternative you could use cultured buttermilk or kefir milk instead. Dairy farmers who produce and sell raw milk usually feed their cows with grass all year long and their cows are healthier to begin with and very clean.

At the turn of the last century, when pasteurization was not available yet, milk cures were known to work wonders with many kinds of illnesses. Today we are taught that raw milk may be contaminated and therefore harmful. Others believe that raw milk with a variety of nutrients and its natural enzymes intact boosts the immune system more than any other food.

One of them is a young man from Chicago. In December of 2008, he decided to campaign for our freedom of choice by going on a forty-day/forty-night bicycle tour through the U.S., living on raw milk and raw milk products only. He gave interviews at different radio stations and intended to bring out a documentary on the benefits of raw milk. During this time, he often slept outdoors without any negative effect on his wellbeing. His wife and two beautiful daughters follow a similar diet. Looking as healthy as he does after overcoming an incurable disease, this young man tries to dissipate the myth that raw milk can be harmful.

Since raw milk is relatively difficult to buy, some clinics suggest regular pasteurized whole milk instead. I tried it and became constipated. The enzymes necessary for good digestion are not present, and as an adult we cannot digest pasteurized milk. It can become a problem. A friend of mine who also followed the Mayr diet with pasteurized milk had the same experience. We then both decided to correct the problem by drinking black cherry juice instead. She followed the program for five to seven weeks and really looked much rejuvenated when I saw her again. The black cherry juice surely sends you to the bathroom, and elimination is the key! We had a good laugh about it.

It is not just the lack of enzymes that makes pasteurized milk inappropriate for human digestion. Apart from the pesticides, antibiotics and growth hormones it might contain, it usually comes homogenized and deodorized, sometimes altered for people who are lactose intolerant and most of the time fat reduced. When you take out the fat, you usually remove magnesium as well, one of the most important minerals for our body. Does it surprise you that pasteurized cow's milk is bad for a calf and can even kill a pet? Additional intake of alkaline minerals may further assist in keeping up your strength. Another option might be to replace the raw milk with either bone broth or rice milk. A variation to the original program is the **New F.X. Mayr Diet**. Starting around the fifth day, one may drink homemade vegetable broth. The broth has extra minerals. After the ninth day, it is permitted to add steamed vegetables and easy to digest proteins like soft cheeses, turkey, ham, or trout. Other supportive measures are abdominal massages, walking, infrared sauna (which is less stressful than the regular sauna), and homeopathic or herbal remedies.

Also, from the second week on, an occasional enema with chamomile tea or a complete colonic irrigation is recommended. Reiki treatments and acupuncture are other methods to increase the body's self healing power. Perhaps the New F.X. Mayr Diet is easier to follow than the original one. The inclusion of lean meat and cooked vegetables helps to ease into a more normal diet. The daily chewing of the white bread and milk still remains the most important part of the cure. So does the daily ingestion of the cleansing drink with Epsom salts in the morning.

Once the program is finished, your follow-up is just as important. Your diet should consist of about 80% alkaline and 20% acid foods. Alkaline foods are: vegetables, fruit (including citrus, which is acid but changes into alkaline), butter, buttermilk as well as raw milk, almonds, seeds and sprouts. Acid forming foods are: bread, pasta, animal protein like meat, fish, eggs, or cheese, coffee and black tea. They should be reduced to a minimum. Neither of the two Mayr diets contains sugar or fat.

Whether you follow the program once a year or during the change of the seasons for renewal, it is always recommended to drink about three quarts of water a day and add minerals in the form of ionic or colloidal supplements. Once you finish the cure, your complexion should have a new glow. Your body shape will be more like the one in your younger years, and your energy (sexual and other) should be like during the best years of your life. Most likely you will experience a noticeable transformation. Best of all, although this is considered a fasting cure, the rolls and the minerals keep you satisfied and you will hardly go hungry the entire time, which makes it easy to follow the program longer and with excellent results.

One of my clients, who is a counselor at a school, was unable to take time off from her busy schedule. She took her milk and hard rolls to the office to chew them there. When the children came in unexpectedly, she explained to them that she was on a special diet and for the time being there were no more candies to be given out. One of the children candidly asked her, "Miss T., is this the Jesus Diet you are on?" She just smiled and thought to herself that it might very well be, because it is supposed to work miracles.

Improve Your Health by Eating Less

Eating is one of our main pleasures. We all love to eat unless we are sick or lose our appetite for some other reason. Eating whatever, whenever, might not have immediate consequences but it is not beneficial in the long run. Our stomach needs an occasional rest.

Not eating at all may be one of the best things we can do for ourselves. In fact, temporary fasting may be the quickest way to return to health. Of course, extremes are not advisable and a better choice may be to either eat less, fewer times during the day, or limit ourselves to very simple, natural foods like fruit. Eating less may be a good way to get the best of both worlds, i.e. to enjoy our meals and be in excellent health as well. There are times when we want to be with friends, eat together and have a good time but in the long run, a little restriction and being more frugal cannot hurt. We can also choose to give our digestive system a complete rest by drinking only water, herbal tea, or fresh juices.

Mono diets are a variation to fasting. We still eat, but limit ourselves to one kind of food only, like apples or grapes. Amber chose to live on fruit only for a whole month. It is difficult, but she reaped tremendous benefits far beyond her physical appearance. Another option may be to eat only salads or brown rice. The Mayr diet is another variation. Whenever we eat small or very simple meals we give our digestive system a rest, and the body uses all its energy to repair and heal itself. Dead and weak cells are eliminated first, and the overall effect will be rejuvenating. Following a mono diet can be challenging. After a while we crave something more palatable but in any case, there will always be benefits. Just by substituting one meal a day for fruit or a green smoothie, can make a noticeable difference.

When people fast with water only, after a day or two, doubts begin to appear. The idea of starvation may come to mind, although more people die from overeating than from temporarily not eating anything at all. Not so with mono diets. We will be hungry, but at least we know that with some food, simple as it may be, we can live a very long time. Even when we live exclusively on fruit, we still get vitamins, some minerals, fiber, and even a little protein. The less we eat, the longer we may live, especially if we choose raw food and chew well.

There is not one program that works for everybody. Nor does the same program work all the time. We have to take into account our environment, climate, social commitments, financial possibilities, and our goals when choosing food and the best time for our meals. After awhile the body gets used to any plan and needs new stimulation. Fortunately, there are a lot of options. One way to find out what works best is through trial and error, and write it down. How do we feel? Does the food give us more energy? Do we feel sluggish? How about gas and stomach cramps? These are all clues as to whether to continue or change to something different.

A good way to find out how to get results is to either ask or observe people who at one time had challenges and then managed to overcome them. Nearly always they are willing to share their stories. I like to observe people at the supermarket. When I get to the cash register, I look at people's faces and compare them to what is in their shopping carts. Usually there is a connection. Young people usually look great and are full of energy, regardless of what they eat. Older people cannot hide what kind of diet they have been following for years. If they filled their carts with packaged foods, white bread, canned goods, cigarettes, meat and cookies they will probably not look like the image of health. They might have a grayish skin tone, are wrinkled ahead of their years, and be out of shape. They may even look sad or bored with life.

If you don't want to resemble them, stay away from the "foods" they consume. A person with fresh produce, nuts, grains, and water bottles in their shopping cart most likely will look different, more energetic, more optimistic, and in better shape. A person advanced in years and who still looks good, probably has a healthy diet. Look at their cart and you will see what makes them beautiful.

Quantity matters as well. It is not the amount of food we ingest but rather the amount of food we absorb and what it does for us. Some eat and eat without adding an ounce to their weight. Overweight people may hardly eat at all and jokingly remark that "even the air makes them fat." The sicker people are, the more often they tend to eat, sometimes three, four, or more meals a day, and the wrong kind of food. Tasty is not always best. Some people get up at night because they are still hungry, craving bread, pasta, sweets, and animal protein. They are more filling, but none of them is health building. Eating all the time leaves residues behind and over time forms a lot of mucus and other build-up in our intestine, thereby creating a perfect breeding ground for parasites.

We do need carbohydrates, vitamins, minerals, some protein, fats, and water. Minerals are particularly important. They are involved in almost every bodily function. We need these nutrients as much as a car needs gasoline. Eating smaller amounts of food or less frequently gives us a chance to eliminate waste more thoroughly. The body will then be in a better position to absorb what it needs. It is important to find a way that is doable and in harmony with your particular lifestyle and which can be maintained over longer periods of time.

Overeating, whether it is in quantity or variety, will make our blood acidic, forming mucus, mold, yeast and fungus. It is not the ideal basis for outstanding health.

By substituting one meal a day with raw food or skipping a meal altogether, we support the body in its cleaning action, and we will soon notice overall improvements. For speedier recovery, it is recommended to eat fruit only one day every week. Dr. Sperl recommended such fruit days every fourth day, and achieved excellent results in all his patients. The practice of not eating anything at all before noon has proven to bring a great variety of health benefits as well, even without the need to make other changes. Each person is different. If you feel hungry in the morning and need to eat eggs, beans, oatmeal or any other kind of protein, you may find it easier to have breakfast and then replace dinner or lunch with a salad or fruit only.

In recent years, a lot of research has been done on anti-aging. We like to live longer and stay youthful. Actually, it is the quality of life that counts, not the amount of years we are around. By eating less, we have a better chance to do so. One of the most effective ways to slow down the aging process is intermittent fasting. It was discovered by Dr. Michael Mosley, a now famous physician from England. It is about alternating periods of eating with those of eating less or nothing at all. The program has become quite popular because people lose weight and become healthier without much effort. It is also called the 5:2 diet and consists of eating normally for five days and reducing our calorie intake the other two days of the week to 500 for women and a maximum of 600-800 calories for men. There is no need to become vegetarian. A friend of mine followed the 5:2 diet and within a few weeks she lost ten pounds. Her husband lost forty pounds within the first year and could get off most of his medication.

A variation would be to reduce our eating time to six to eight hours and not eat more than two meals a day. We may skip one meal completely, which can be breakfast, lunch, or dinner. Beauty expert and author Tonya Zavasta recommends eating in the morning and a second meal later. She consumes no food or water after 2:00 p.m. and looks stunning. Muslims during the holy month of Ramadan eat one meal before the sun comes up and another one after the sun goes down, with no food or water in between. These alternatives are effective, but not easy to follow for the average person, especially over longer periods of time.

Whenever we eat less and more natural food, we give Mother Nature a chance to restore health, sometimes in advanced cases when medical doctors are at a loss. She promptly responds to any changes we make. Although we might soon see improvements, disease and premature aging did not happen overnight. It might require some patience and consistency to reverse them. Fasting and reduced eating are some of the most powerful processes we have access to. Although physicians may give us assistance, we are the ones to lay the groundwork. We need to get rid of toxic matter.

Henry's Transformation

My friend and mentor Henry was a beautiful person, kind, peaceful, compassionate, and the image of good health. He was a most remarkable man teaching from his own experience. Originally, he was from Spain. We met in Mexico City when I was at the beginning of my path to health and chose to become vegetarian. Henry was much older than I. He had blue eyes, was relatively slim, and all year round had a nice golden tan. There was a radiance about him, which made people want to be close to him.

I met Henry at one of the upscale vegetarian restaurants in Mexico City. He was a bachelor and never cooked for himself. So he had his lunch and sometimes also supper at the restaurant. Everybody seemed to know him. He was well liked and his cheerful personality made it easy to talk to him. Usually, he sat by himself, enjoying his meals in silence. He always looked happy, grateful, as if God personally had served him this day a very special meal and he had much to be thankful for. Henry became one of my best friends. He was always willing to answer questions and help me over the next hurdle when I was about to get discouraged with many a healing crisis.

I was on Dr. Sperl's diet at the time and still had my doubts whether going on a vegetarian diet was going to work for me. Sometimes I seemed to get worse instead of better. I had stomach cramps, painful gas, and my skin broke out with blemishes. It was not until years later, and thanks to Henry's patience, that I understood these reactions were part of my recovery. My body was trying to free itself from previously prescribed medicine and other toxins. Looking at Henry, who had been on this path much longer than I had, was quite an encouragement. I was so glad I could ask him questions.

Henry was indeed the image of good health. He must have been in his fifties at that time, but had no wrinkles at all. It was hard to guess his age. He always had a nice smile on his face. One day he shared his story about how it all started for him. Henry (Enrique) grew up in Spain. As a young man, he was terribly, terribly sick. His father owned a candy factory and a tobacco store, something he considered a blessing. He loved chocolates and liked to smoke cigarettes. Not having to pay for them made him consume more than was good for him. He also shared some of them with his friends, whom he met in different bars in the evening.

Henry's generosity made him quite popular with the other guys. At home, his meals consisted of meat, fish, desserts, and white bread, usually accompanied by a bottle of wine. In the evenings he ate out, enjoying ham and sausages and some alcohol at a bar. This went on for quite some time, until one day he was so sick he could not get out of bed. His usual good appetite for "delicacies" was gone. He felt a terrible weakness and started vomiting. His mother called several doctors to figure out what was wrong with him. None of the medicines seemed to help. Henry remembered just lying there, for days, unable to get up. He could not eat anything, except for some fruit. Apparently, this made him feel better.

As soon as he could get up, he went back to the bars and his old ways. When he got sick again, he decided to try the fruit thing again. Again, much to his surprise, it seemed to help rather quickly. He went back to the bars with his usual diet of meat, candies, cigarettes, and alcohol in moderation. After awhile he thought he knew the answer. Whenever he got sick, he would eat fruit. Down went his health and he ate fruit again. He recovered and returned to junk, getting sick again. After a while, he was able to recognize a pattern: Whenever he lived on nothing but fruit, his health quickly returned and he felt better, whereas his usual diet of meat, fine desserts, unlimited amounts of candies, cigarettes, and alcohol had a devastating effect on him. Although he was only in his twenties at the time, Henry felt more than once that he was close to dying, at least this was how miserable he felt. As a result of these abuses, he lost his hair and quite a few teeth at an early age.

Eventually, he got sick of feeling sick and tired and looking older than his age. He started including more fruit and salads in his diet. He dropped some of his vices and enjoyed feeling good more often. He then made up his mind to become vegetarian. After reading books on health and the benefits of raw food, he decided to throw away all his pots and frying pans. Later on, he added soups and some cooked vegetables at the restaurant. This was a major turning point in his life. His health improved dramatically and he never had to worry about it again. Henry told me that when he changed his eating habits his whole life changed. His old friends were not his friends anymore. He met new people with similar interests. He changed his profession to photographer and spent much of his time in nature observing the beauty of flowers and birds. He also started meditating. I got the impression he was something like a saint, always kind and generous to everybody, and he had a wonderful sense of humor.

One day he mentioned that he had read about the healing power of garlic. He decided to eat as much as he could, which were about twenty-eight cloves in one day, and then he left his house to see a movie. Henry got into a taxi cab and had just traveled a few blocks, when the driver stopped the car and opened the door. He asked Henry politely to get out immediately and either walk or look for another vehicle because the smell was more than he could bear. We all had a good laugh at his story and realized what can happen if you take things to an extreme.

The Invisible Danger: Parasites!

Any cleansing or rejuvenating diet can work wonders and may bring about surprising results. However, sometimes these kinds of diets, no matter how simple they may be, might be difficult to follow due to uninvited guests called parasites who keep claiming their share.

Parasites range in size and form, and they all have one thing in common: they love to eat. They look for nutrients in our body and then leave their waste, keeping us constantly tired and hungry. You may still feel hungry after a meal because you actually don't get the nutrients you are eating. The parasites get them! Once you are free from these little scavengers, you will notice that your appetite diminishes. Your body starts to absorb the food better, strengthening you and not your enemies.

When we think of parasites, we might relate them to people in third world countries, poor hygiene, children who don't wash their hands, or infested drinking water. It may never occur to us that anybody in a clean environment might get infested as well. In fact, it is estimated that over 80 percent of the population in the United States have some form of parasites, ranging from microscopically small ones to those several feet long.

Some of them are not easily detected and may cause health challenges like constipation, diarrhea, a weak immune system, joint and muscle aches and pains, mineral deficiencies, gas and bloating, allergies, breathing problems, cough, skin conditions, sleep disturbances, tooth grinding, lack of energy, mood swings, excess weight, heart and circulatory problems, and many others. Currently, there are over one hundred kinds of known parasites and only about 20 percent of them tend to show up in conventional stool tests. Although small in size, they can be so dangerous in the long run that some experts refer to them as "the silent killers."

Once they have found a human host, parasites can lay thousands of eggs a day. These travel in our blood stream and can go into any organ of the body and multiply there, devouring nutrients first and then leaving their waste. Allergies or continuous coughing may be a sign of parasites in our lungs and bronchial area. The body tries to remove the invaders and their waste in the form of mucus or phlegm. As long as parasites are present, the body is unable to fully recuperate due to a lack of vitamins and minerals. Medication will temporarily control the symptoms, and diets alone take much longer to work than when combined with special herbs to get rid of the parasites.

If the immune system stays weak, and not all eggs and larvae are removed, they hatch later and start a new cycle. More effective ways to detect the presence of even the smallest kind of parasites than stool analysis is kinesiology (muscle testing), dowsing, or dark field blood analysis. These methods are practiced by natural healers and are not found in a traditional clinical environment.

The first question people ask after being made aware of the possibility that they might have parasites is "How did I get them?" They exist in fruit, vegetables, raw meat, especially pork, in the water we drink; we can get them by touching a pet or walking barefoot, handling money, coming in contact with door handles, keys and other objects. They can also be transmitted from one family member to another. In other words: Parasites are everywhere! This does not necessarily mean we get them. If we have a strong immune system, our body deals with them and knows how to eliminate them. It is only when our immune system has been compromised due to stress, illness, or medication that it cannot deal with these often-invisible enemies and needs help. Once the parasites are gone, a variety of symptoms disappear on their own.

A Spanish physician who eventually changed his career to naturopathy, told the story of one of his patients who had been diagnosed with intestinal cancer. She was scheduled for surgery to have part of her colon removed due to a large "tumor." The young woman was absolutely frightened at the thought of having to wear a bag for waste removal for the rest of her life and begged the doctor for an alternative solution. He offered her a program consisting of nutritional changes in combination with certain herbs. A few weeks later, she telephoned him, all excited, and told him that she had just expelled what seemed to be the tumor. She then asked him if he wanted her to bring the stuff to the office for examination. He suggested she have it analyzed in a lab and then let him know about the results. It turned out that what she expelled was not a tumor, but a large cyst of parasites. Needless to say, her surgery was cancelled.

The danger of parasites is that they mimic other diseases, and instead of going to the root of the problem, most doctors keep treating symptoms whereas the real cause is ignored. The microscopically small ones are the most dangerous ones. They tend to suck the life out of their hosts. Parasites love food. They can exist in waste material, but enjoy especially mucus forming foods, like milk and dairy products. Sugar is another of their favorites. Therefore, cravings might be due to parasites!

Since they multiply more readily in an impacted colon, constipation may be the number one cause for their existence. Of course, anything that is good for the host is also good for parasites. Therefore, one should be careful before taking vitamins and minerals. Guess who gets to eat them first! If they lay 8,000 eggs a day, just imagine how fertile the parasites may become with extra vitamins. Therefore, most nutritional supplements should not be taken until a cleansing has taken place and you are sure that all harmful microorganisms have been removed. Otherwise, you strengthen the enemy instead of yourself.

Parasites are relatively easy to get rid of with anti-parasite herbs and colon cleansing products. Since a majority of people do have parasites without being aware of them as the cause of their symptoms, you might wonder if it is a good idea to go on an anti-parasitic program just in case. In countries like Mexico, where nearly everybody suffers from dangerous amoeba and other types of parasites, the Department of Health recommends that the population undergo a regular de-worming program at least once a year. The problem is that those medications are rather strong. Although they kill off parasites, they may also affect body tissues making the host each time more susceptible to new invasions.

Also, the parasites themselves are becoming more resistant to drugs. Are there other options? If you suspect you have parasites and do not have access to a health practitioner who uses any of the above mentioned natural methods to detect unwanted critters in your body or just as a general preventative measure, you might decide to buy an herbal combination at a health food store especially designed to eliminate parasites. Different brands are available, also over the internet. Most of these products are gentle and can be taken without side effects. Often, they contain clove, garlic, pumpkin seeds, or wormwood.

Such herbs do not harm your body, but are greatly detested by parasites. One could say they make life miserable for them, so they opt to leave the body. Some herbal formulas come in combination with a bowel cleanser which also helps to expel unwanted microorganisms and keeps the colon clean. A clean colon with sufficient beneficial bacteria offers neither food nor shelter for parasites. You may repeat the process once a year, or as soon as you suspect they are back.

Signs may be itching of the eyes, nose or rectal area, frequent coughing or low energy. Of course, it is best to be tested first. If no parasites are present, then there is no point in taking a product for something you don't have. However, if you want to cleanse yourself in a preventative way, or because you suspect you might have uninvited guests in your body, then a natural cleanser is best. Also, it is a good idea to try different brands, since the ingredients of one product may be more effective for you than others.

If at all possible, take enemas or go for a colonic in the beginning of your self-treatment to speed up the process. One might see worms coming out, alive or dead. Another sign of their presence may be a foul smell due to the gas they release when they die off. You might never see parasites coming out, but by the way you look and feel afterwards you can tell that they have disappeared. You feel clean. No more gas or bloating, and your overall energy increases tremendously.

One Cause, A Thousand Disguises

If there is anything worse than having parasites it is having a dangerous fungal overgrowth called Candida or Candidiasis, mainly because it can be present for years without causing pain and is difficult to detect.

Candida normally resides in our body. It can be in our mouth, throat, intestines and the genitourinary tract. If it is kept in check, there is no danger. However, once our friendly bacteria have been reduced, Candida converts into a fungus, ready to invade other organs. It is the most undetected cause of nearly all disease and it can become deadly. When we think of killer diseases, what comes to mind is cancer, AIDS and heart problems. Hardly anybody thinks of yeast or fungus as a killer and yet, an estimated 95 percent of the U.S. population suffer from Candida overgrowth as a **cause** of these and many other serious illnesses.

Candida albicans, as it is called, is a normal part of our intestinal flora, which makes up about 80 percent of our immune system. A healthy person has a properly functioning immune system with mostly good bacteria. When these are destroyed, our immune system becomes weakened and Candida proliferates. It can then affect every organ of our body. Some of the most common symptoms are weight gain, insomnia, low energy and cravings for sweets or bread with yeast in it. Good intestinal bacteria can be killed off with antibiotics, hormones, toxic metals (such as mercury found in dental fillings), any form of radiation, anesthesia, cortisone, most vaccines and even chlorine in tap water. Excessive stress or hormone imbalances may also create an overgrowth of the fungus.

Candida can invade any organ of the body. Going into the brain it can cause depression, anxiety or nervousness. It can affect the liver, which is involved in an estimated 200 to 500 functions, including the formation of cholesterol and triglycerides. It can affect our lungs and bronchia. It can go into our sexual organs causing infertility and endometriosis in women and sexual dysfunction in men. It can affect every cell and still remain undetected. It does not cause any pain although it may be a cause for cancer, heart and circulatory issues.

It may cause AIDS, lupus, arthritis, MS, diabetes, and so many others. It can destroy teeth and bones. If left unrecognized and untreated, a person may die from it, especially if it hits the brain. Some physicians call it the disease in a thousand disguises although it is not a disease but rather their **cause.** Others deny its existence. It is hard to detect with conventional methods and physicians rather treat the symptoms. Just as cancer cells, the presence of Candida does not cause pain. It feeds on sugar and some doctors believe both are the same. Of course, there are different degrees. Some people are more affected than others.

There are over 150 strains of Candida, all difficult to detect in lab tests. Candida cells attach to the mucus lining inside the body and hardly ever show up in a stool analysis. It may present itself as a hormone imbalance, as thyroid malfunction, dry skin, impotence, hypoglycemia, diabetes, bad breath, bloating, gas, constipation or diarrhea, dry mouth, obesity, acne, blurred vision, mineral deficiency, bone loss, chest pain, hay fever, head pain, brain fog, migraines, allergies, muscle aches, numbness, sinus problems, lupus, psoriasis, excessive perspiration, nail fungus, bladder infection, cramps, endometriosis, irregular or painful menstruation, water retention, infertility, loss of sexual feelings, painful intercourse, itching or discharge, asthma, breathing problems, arthritis, anxiety, tooth loss, insomnia, high blood pressure, depression, dry eyes, anxiety, attention deficit, cancer, weakness, poor memory, lupus, MS, mottled skin, discolorations, weight problems, cold hands and feet, or others. In other words, Candida may be the cause of any and all disease. Getting rid of it can initiate the return to health in most cases.

Candida poisons the bloodstream and prevents the absorption of oxygen and important nutrients. The symptoms vary from one patient to the next, which is another reason why nobody suspects that the cause is the same for all of them. One patient may be treated for arthritis, another one has diabetes, another one tumors, infertility or depression, depending on the organ or areas of the body which are affected. The underlying cause may be the same for all of them.

I am neither a medical doctor nor a scientist, so I have no idea what Candida exactly looks like inside the body. Some describe it as something white that you may or may not see in your stools. Others say it forms root-like structures. Another enigma is that the fungus may attach to perfectly healthy organs and cause them to malfunction. It can affect the heart, the bones, or the thyroid gland among others. Once the fungus is eliminated, the body goes back to functioning normal again and starts to heal itself.

Dr. Tullio Simoncini, a famous Italian oncologist who also specializes in diabetes and other metabolic disorders, published a book entitled *Cancer is a Fungus*, in which he describes his scientific findings. He concluded that Candida is the basis for all cancers as well as the cause of diabetes and many other degenerative diseases. His observations are that it spreads inside the body causing tumors and tissue alterations. He is of the opinion that chemotherapy and radiation, two of the most conventional treatments for cancer, cause an increase in Candida and, therefore, do not restore the body to health. Although he healed many people of so-called incurable diseases, mainly by administrating baking soda orally and by injection, he and his treatments are shunned by the medical profession.

The late Dr. William Crook went so far as to say that **Candida is practically the cause of every disease,** especially those of a chronic or degenerative nature. He has written several books on the subject, including *The Candida Connection*.

Although it is estimated that over 95 percent of Americans suffer from an overgrowth of Candida, the sad truth is that hardly anybody is aware of it. Doctors do not mention it. It can affect men, women, and children in the most terrible way or ...... present no symptoms at all for years and go undetected. Sometimes the only symptoms are low energy or being overweight, both of which can be attributed to other factors. As long as Candida is present, true healing will not be possible.

In fact, it is mostly medical procedures that cause Candida. Even a visit to the dentist, which includes X-rays and anesthesia, is not without danger and can cause systemic Candida. So, what is the way out when we absolutely need those procedures? The best option may be to follow an anti-Candida diet, avoiding sugar as much as possible and taking probiotics. It may take days, weeks, or even months before symptoms show up, and they may remain totally unrelated to their original cause.

The main danger is that it does not cause pain and may remain undetected for years. Medication to treat the symptoms may cause additional damage and sometimes the problems become irreversible. How can we know whether an overgrowth of Candida is present? One way is to specifically request a test from your doctor. Another, not very scientific, possibility is to have a glass of water next to your bed and first thing in the morning spit in it. If the saliva forms legs in the water, Candida is present. Other tests are based on energy. Although they are mostly used by natural healers only, they are quite reliable. Such tests include kinesiology (muscle testing), radio-aesthesia (dowsing) and dark field blood analysis. Just by looking at a person's skin one can sometimes tell that there is a possibility of Candida. When it is dry, red, blotchy, mottled, cracked, has sore spots, shows moles or wart-like growths, tags, or feels very itchy most likely there is an overgrowth. These skin alterations can show up on the face, arms, neck, scalp, hands or feet and usually do not heal or change. They can also appear as fungus on toe and fingernails. When treated with medication, the fungus might be killed off temporarily, but it will come back in a more resistant form. To make things worse, parasites are often present simultaneously. The symptoms are similar and, therefore, difficult to differentiate unless you do energy testing or see either one under a dark field microscope.

According to Dr. Simoncini, cancer is always an overgrowth of Candida and healing can only take place when its cause is corrected and not by cutting off organs or damaging the body in any other way. Although we can live without certain organs, it does not mean that we do not need them. Each surgery puts more stress on the remaining organs and there is a greater possibility for them to eventually break down as well.

The most effective way to restore balance in our digestive system is through a change in diet in combination with targeted natural products and probiotics. Anything sweet, fermented, or with yeast in it must be avoided until you get rid of the fungus. Foods like bread, cakes, cheese, soft drinks, wine, vinegar, sweet fruit, and alcohol accelerate its growth. Candida does not distinguish between good sugar and refined sugar. It simply feeds on anything sweet. Fruits permitted without causing further harm are apples, pears, papaya, kiwi, berries, plums, and limes or lemons. No oranges or grapefruit either! No commercial salad dressing or ketchup is allowed during a Candida treatment, since it contains vinegar and sugar. Although yogurt and fruit in general are considered healthy foods, they perpetuate the problem. These "forbidden" foods are exactly the ones we crave most when an excess of Candida is present. Apart from sugar, the fungus loves bread, cakes, cheese, and alcohol.

It is possible to have Candidiasis for ten, twenty or more years without being aware of it. The problem has become rampant in the U.S. due to the increased use of antibiotics and other drugs. Other causes may be vaccinations and X-rays. Preferably ask for a pat-down at the airport. There may be no detectible symptoms for a very long time or only a few painless ones like weight gain, low energy, insomnia, tooth decay, or cravings for sweets, bread or alcohol. However, over time, the desire for sugar and alcohol may become irresistible.

With proper diet, especially the total avoidance of sugar in any form, and certain supplements, Candida can be brought under control relatively fast, and the overgrowth can be eliminated within a matter of weeks. Once the fungus is gone, so will the cravings. Most of the other symptoms will disappear as well. People then start losing weight easily regardless of the amount of food they eat. Their energy comes back. They sleep better and regain their positive outlook on life. People return to health.

While on a Candida diet, vegetables in any form are highly recommended. Protein and fats are fine too. So are nuts, potatoes, rice, corn tortillas and flat breads without yeast. Milk and dairy products must be avoided. Among animal proteins, fish is the most recommended, since it contains plenty of minerals. Fowl, eggs, and red meat are okay. One can also eat all kinds of fat, nuts, beans and lentils. Oriental diets with rice, vegetables, and a little meat are ideal. Leafy green vegetables alkalize our blood and are among the most healing foods we can eat. Taking probiotics is highly recommended to restore the balance of the intestinal flora.

Other excellent supplements are fresh garlic, colloidal silver, Pau D'arco tea, grapefruit seed and olive leaf extract. The most powerful herb in fighting Candida is fresh garlic. It is recommended to ingest a clove of raw garlic at least once a day. It can be chopped up and then swallowed with a glass of water to which some lime or lemon juice has been added. The lemon juice takes care of the smell.

How do you know you got rid of the fungus? First of all, you will feel different. Your energy will increase, your mind will be clearer, you may lose weight without effort, and you will sleep better, not to mention that other conditions will disappear. Sugar cravings will also diminish. You can do the spit test again and observe if there are any legs formed by the saliva.

Once the fungus is gone, protein consumption should be somewhat reduced. Fruit and natural sweeteners like stevia or raw honey may be consumed again in moderation. You may also eat whole grain bread, preferably toasted, some cheese (preferably from raw milk), and have an occasional glass of wine. Eating garlic on a regular basis protects you and keeps your energy up. If "an apple a day keeps the doctor away," taking a clove of garlic a day is probably even more powerful and helps you stay out of the doctor's office.

Eat Rice for Youthfulness

In Western countries we believe that the best diets include lots of fruit and vegetables, meat, and some carbohydrates from bread, potatoes, rice or pasta and that it is a good idea to avoid salt and sugar.

We believe that to stay in shape it is important to reduce our fat intake and count calories. In Asia, people value the concept of balance, and the perfect food to achieve it is rice as a staple. For thousands of years they have been eating rice, steamed vegetables, sea weeds, and fish. Maybe it is a diet that helps to stay young. Orientals tend to have a longer life span and a more peaceful attitude. Cancer and heart problems, the number one and two killer diseases in the U.S., are rare. Whether it is the rice itself that promotes youthfulness is hard to tell. Genes could be part of it, or the fact that Asians avoid many food items that promote disease and premature aging, especially refined sugar and its substitutes. They consume less animal protein, hardly any milk and dairy products, packaged foods, bread with yeast or pastry.

When we compare ourselves to people in countries where rice is eaten almost daily, it is surprising how young and slim they look. People in Asian countries hardly have wrinkles, especially around the eye area, and their hair stays dark to an advanced age. In Japan, for instance, until recently it was hard to even find chocolate, dairy products, or pastries for sale. There was not much demand for them by the natives. Rice, vegetables and a little animal protein keep them strong and healthy, and those foods seem to be beneficial for all human beings. White, refined sugar is hardly consumed in Asian countries. Sugar may produce a temporary high, but at the same time it depletes our body of nutrients and actually lowers our energy reserves. Besides, it is addictive.

I never realized how addicted I was to sugar until I visited Japan. After a few days without access to anything sweet, fermented or with yeast in it, I felt miserable. Being vegetarian at the time, I thought I had a good diet with a lot of fruit in it and occasional candy bars. Searching for something more appropriate for my taste buds, I located a tiny grocery store where they carried a piece of cheese and some cookies. The cheese was old and the cookies tasted awful. Apparently, they had been there a while. The locals preferred rice, fish and vegetables.

In some areas of India and in Japan, fresh fruit can only be bought by the rich. At least in the past it was considered a rare delicacy, only eaten sparingly, partly because it was expensive and sometimes hard to come by. Poor people could not afford to buy much animal protein and fruit, and in general they were much healthier.

In 1990, the price for a single melon in Japan was $300 US. I took a picture of a melon with the price tag on it because compared to Mexico, where fruit is abundant and melons at the time only cost less than a dollar each, it was an exorbitant price. More recent research seems to confirm that sweet fruit is not the health food we believed it to be. It contains lots of sugar and very few minerals. Bread and cakes baked with yeast are not very health promoting either. In many parts of Asia, Africa and South America, people eat flat bread without yeast. They prefer the flat bread, like corn tortillas in Mexico, because the oven baked bread with yeast makes them feel bloated. The Bible* also mentions the importance of eating unleavened bread.

An acquaintance of mine told me that her mother-in-law looked extremely young in spite of her age and the fact that she ate almost anything. I asked her if there was anything special in her diet that she ate or did not eat that kept her so young. She thought about it for a moment and then replied that the only thing her mother-in-law never ate was anything with yeast in it. Maybe there is wisdom in avoiding it. People with Candida will definitely benefit and thrive on a diet of rice and vegetables, without sugar, dairy, and fermented foods.

Sakurazawa Nyoiti, or George Ohsawa (1893-1966), as he was known in the West, and founder of macrobiotics, came up with a diet which was deemed to be most healing even after other diets had failed. He considered brown rice, vegetables and sea salt the perfect food for health and longevity, mainly because of its ideal ratio of 5:1 between potassium and sodium, giving the body the perfect balance between yin and yang energies. Brown rice contains fiber, some minerals, and valuable vitamins of the B complex. He believed that living for ten days exclusively on brown rice and herbal tea was enough to change the body's chemistry.

He also praised the healing qualities of all vegetables, which could be added later on, and suggested that sugar, dairy, yeast, and fruit, with the exception of cherries, apples and strawberries in very small amounts, should be avoided completely. He also believed in the need to consume unrefined sea salt for its mineral content. His program became known as macrobiotics, "macro" meaning great and "bio" meaning life. His ten-day brown rice diet became popular in the sixties, especially in the USA and France, where Mr. Ohsawa had many followers. Although, later on, his diet was criticized due to its lack of other nutrients, it helped many people to return to health after they had been given up by their doctors.

Mr. Ohsawa believed it was his brown rice diet, combined with daily exercise, that brought him back to life after suffering from an "incurable" disease in his younger years. The most famous book on his work, translated into English, is *You are all Sampaku* (*Sick*). He believes that ten days on brown rice only are sufficient for almost any kind of health challenge. This is the time span for our blood cells to renew themselves completely. He believes that at a rate of 300 million globules per second, or one tenth of the total amount each day, our blood can be entirely renewed within ten days.

The first time I heard about this diet was when I was teaching yoga classes in the Northern part of Mexico. One of my students, a beautiful lady in her late seventies, mentioned it to me. Despite her age, she was amazingly flexible and had a youthful complexion. I was surprised to see her bend her legs over her shoulders in one of the positions, just as I did, although she was forty years my senior. She said that she attributed her looks and flexibility to the ten-day rice diet, which she had followed years earlier. She believed it had helped her to lose weight and made her complexion so clear and rosy that she became the belle of the ball in her time. Fortunately, she was willing to share whatever she remembered about the diet, so I could try it myself.

I followed the diet for the entire ten days, which was not easy. I lost so much weight that even my shoes became too big. Although this is not a favorite of mine, I admit that my hair and skin looked much better after the ten days. My weight returned to normal as soon as I added more liquids again and I felt very good afterwards, more energetic, and my concentration improved as well. Using fermented rice like GABA or soaking the rice overnight may give even better results. GABA (short for gamma amino butyric acid) rice, is whole grain sprouted brown rice. It is supposed to be the healthiest form of rice. It is gluten free and non-allergenic. The germination process itself adds a variety of nutrients and activates dormant enzymes.

The original ten-day diet as recommended by Mr. Ohsawa is as follows:

Bring to boil one cup of brown rice with with two cups of water and a teaspoonful of unrefined sea salt. After five minutes, lower the heat and let the rice simmer for approximately one hour. It gives the daily portion for each of the ten days. Liquid is only allowed sparingly with about two cups of herbal or green tea a day.

After the ten days, one may add vegetables, soups, and some protein like fish, fowl, or eggs to the brown rice. Dairy products, sugar, and yeast should be avoided for good. The effects on hair, skin, and weight are noticeable even before the ten days are over. Several friends of mine tried the diet for seven to ten days and loved the benefits, but they also found it difficult to follow. My own advice would be to drink more than two cups of tea, especially if you live in a hot climate.

* You can alternate the brown rice with carrot juice and drink herbal tea as often as desired;
* If you need something juicy, eat a few apples in between your portions of rice.
* Adding Chia seeds and drinking more tea improves bowel movements. Rice tends to cause constipation in some people.

It is amazing what drinking green tea and eating rice and vegetables can do for a person's complexion. On one occasion, I visited a Chinese restaurant with a girlfriend. The waiter had the most amazingly beautiful skin. It was rosy, with not even one tiny little wrinkle. After several trips to the buffet, my friend and I debated whether we should ask him about his secret. Most likely he was not using any beauty creams, so it must be something else. Finally, we got the courage to bring it up.

He was very open about it and, smiling, he said it was nothing special. He had been eating rice and vegetables every day at the buffet since he worked at the restaurant and drank green tea, lots of it. We asked him how much green tea, to which he replied: a lot, maybe twenty cups a day. He was referring to Chinese cups, which are smaller and would make about ten to twelve regular sized cups.

Another form to eat rice and vegetables is in the form of "kitchari" as it is called in India. Kitchari is a tasty mixture of rice and vegetables with spices added to it. There are different ways to prepare it. One way is to boil either brown or basmati rice for about twenty to thirty minutes, then add mung beans and vegetables like peas, carrots, celery, green beans, broccoli, or cauliflower, and let everything simmer for another ten minutes. You can add ghee or coconut oil, and spices like coriander, cumin seed, turmeric, fresh cilantro, and mineral salt to taste. Some Ayurvedic practitioners believe that if eaten long enough, kitchari heals almost any disease.

Adding chia or hemp seeds to a rice dish may have extra benefits. Chia seed was a diet staple of the Aztecs and Mayans in Mexico. It is believed to have numerous medicinal benefits and is a powerhouse of nutrients. Chia acts as a mild laxative, which is convenient when mixed with cooked rice. These tiny seeds contain alpha-linoleic acid (ALA), as well as calcium, iron, magnesium, some protein and healthy fats. Hemp seeds have similar benefits. The owner of a shelled hemp seed company says that in 1995 he weighed over 300 pounds, was unhealthy and unhappy, and that hemp foods changed his life. Not only did he lose weight, he also got enough energy to climb a mountain for the first time in his life. Convinced of the benefits, he started his own company, hoping to help others experience positive changes as well.

Knowing that at least 75 percent of the world's population, especially Asians, eat rice every day and look wonderful, I believe that rice, especially brown rice, has rejuvenating effects. It may not contain the full spectrum of nutrients, but you can add other items to your diet to make it more palatable. Experience has shown that rice eaters from all over the world look relatively young all their life.

Fasting as a Fountain of Youth

Whenever we eat, the body uses a great deal of its energy for digestion. The less we eat, the more energy the body has available for repair and rejuvenation. The most powerful healing method is to temporarily abstain from food altogether. During a fast, the body produces HGH (Human Growth Hormone), the hormone that keeps us flexible, energetic, and more like we used to be in our earlier years. Old, dead, weak, and diseased cells are being removed and then gradually replaced with new tissue. Fasting is a powerful tool to extend our life span and regain youthfulness. All religions recommend it, because apart from physical improvements, it brings spiritual benefits as well. The Bible* refers to fasting over seventy times. The process has also been called "the surgeon operating without a knife."

There are several ways to fast, the most drastic one being water fasting, where you consume nothing but water. A step further is dry fasting, where you neither eat nor drink anything at all. Its followers say that they live on cosmic energy only. It is probably not something one can keep up very long because otherwise we will literally soon "become one with the earth," and that is not our purpose, at least not ahead of time. Then there is juice fasting, which is self-explanatory, or the kind where you temporarily give up certain foods like meat or sugar. It is sometimes practiced by Christians during Lent.

If you ever intentionally skipped a meal, you know that fasting or semi-fasting requires discipline. You may also remember the initial hunger pangs if you tried to abstain from food for more than a day. During such time, the body eliminates toxins and there may also be tiredness, low energy, bad breath, headaches, feeling irritable or a sense of boredom. Fasting is something like a thorough house cleaning. Being in a sociable environment makes it even harder to resist temptations. Then there is the fear of the unknown.

If you decide to live on water only for several days, the question of starving to death may come to mind. Actually, one is more likely to die from overeating than from fasting, but there are no guarantees. The best way to try it out is to start very slowly by skipping one meal a day. Then you might want to eat only fruit for a whole day. After that, when you realize nothing terrible happens, on the contrary, the next day you feel a lot better than you did before, then you might try an entire day drinking only water. Most people say that they feel better after they don't eat.

My own experience is that I always felt hungry and sometimes low in energy while fasting. An alternative to water fasting is juice fasting, where we still get some nutrients as well as enzymes and a little fiber. Keeping our food intake to a minimum and temporarily avoiding fat, protein, and sugar is another possibility, but it is not really considered fasting.

In his documentary, *Fat, Sick and Nearly Dead*, Joe Cross describes his odyssey living on nothing but fruit and vegetable juices for two months. Joe became an inspiration to many due to the results he achieved. He started out at 420 pounds and had so many health challenges that his doctor told him he would not be around very long unless he changed his eating habits. He lost about 100 pounds on his juice fast under medical supervision. He kept juicing afterwards and now looks athletic, vibrantly healthy, and has a glowing complexion. In combination with his diet, Joe also walked and exercised every day. He keeps on juicing and feels and looks much younger than when he started. He wrote several books on the benefits of juicing.

Most of us do not suffer from life-threatening diseases, but there are signs of aging which can be eliminated with fasting or semi-fasting, like being overweight, vision problems, poor memory, wrinkles, eczema, age spots, loss of libido, toenail fungus, rigidity of joints, depression or low energy, just to mention a few. Nowadays, many of these symptoms are so common they are considered a normal part of the aging process. They can be reversed if we are willing to do our part. The Bible* (Deut. 34:7) says that Moses was a hundred and twenty years old when he died and his eyes were not dim nor was his natural vigor diminished. In other words, he was healthy up to the last day. He fasted for forty days and we can assume that in Biblical times people ate much less than we do today. They certainly did not eat three meals a day, sometimes not even once every day. In our times, there are also individuals who believe in the outstanding benefits of fasting or eating very little to remain youthful.

Author and artist Markus Rothkranz and his partner Cara Brotman are proof of it. Markus in his fifties looks younger than he did twenty or thirty years ago. Markus at one time fasted for forty days in the desert. Both Markus and Cara follow a raw food diet alternating with fasting and exercise.

Fasting remains the number one recipe for rejuvenation, no matter what the problem may be. Even our addictions to certain foods are easier to overcome after a day of fasting or at least reducing our food intake considerably. The ideal may be eating only one meal a day. Elijah Muhammad (1897–1975), a Black American religious leader, who described himself as a messenger of the Prophet Mohammed, in his book *How to Eat to Live* stresses the importance of eating only once every twenty-four hours as the best way to stay or get healthy. He and his followers had a religious center in Arizona, and anybody who met them confirmed that all of them looked very youthful. Whether one could live 500 years this way, as they claimed, is another matter.

True yogis, who are known for their endurance, wisdom, and longevity, also fast periodically. Eating less, or nothing at all, for a certain time might lead to an extended life span, mental clarity, and more vitality. Often it is not until our later years that we achieve our greatest success in life. We would miss out on a lot by not being around anymore. Great actors, scientists, politicians, business people and artists like Picasso, Michelangelo, Pablo Casals, and Verdi seem to prove it.

The German Chancellor Konrad Adenauer (1876-1967) lived a long and frugal life, tending his roses as a hobby in his spare time. He served as Chancellor for so many years that people joked about it. They say that when Adenauer was over ninety years old, he asked his great-grandson what he wanted to become when he grew up. The little guy answered, "Chancellor, grandpa, like you." Adenauer replied that that was impossible because the position was already taken by him and also would be in the future to come. Not all these famous successful people are known to have fasted, but some of them certainly lived a frugal life.

One of these incredible people is a man by the name of Fauja Singh. In April of 2012, he ran a marathon in London at the age of 101. It was his eighth marathon, and he finished the twenty-six miles in seven hours and forty-nine minutes, becoming the oldest man mentally and physically able to ever run a marathon. Mr. Singh did not start running before he was in his eighties. Most people, if still alive being over 100 years old, would probably be crippled and in a nursing home. At the end of the marathon, Mr. Singh was asked about his outstanding condition. With the help of an interpreter, he replied that he attributed it to his simple lifestyle. He said he did not take any medication nor had he ever undergone any surgeries. He said that he only ate small portions, more like a child's portion, and that he drank plenty of tea. He claimed that being stress-free and having a cheerful attitude was also important. People who saw him running said that he had been smiling during the whole marathon.

Another person who attributes his transformation to fasting is a man living in a prison cell. Some eighteen years back he committed a crime under the influence of alcohol. When he entered the prison, he suffered from serious health challenges but according to him it was also where his transformation began physically, spiritually, and mentally. He started meditating frequently and read books on the lives and teachings of spiritual masters. Now, at fifty-eight, he is healthy and his visitors say that he looks more like thirty-five or forty.

When asked how the changes occurred, he believes that fasting may have contributed to it. Initially, he fasted one day a week on water only and then changed to five consecutive days at the beginning of each month. Other contributing factors may have been his practice of meditation and physical work in the fields. When asked about his former health challenges, he said that all his life he had problems with alcohol and that his soul was asleep. When he arrived at the U.S. prison they detected serious liver damage. His whole body was intoxicated. At times, he thought he had cancer because he felt so bad. His bones were aching. He felt dizzy, had high blood pressure, irregular heartbeat, and pain all over. He remembers that his kidneys and his lower back were hurting and that his feet and knees were swollen. His thoughts were not of a positive nature either. At times, he felt so miserable that he considered suicide. However, something inside never abandoned him and started guiding him towards his higher good. With all his physical pain and mental anguish, he started to fast and gradually began to detoxify his body. He tried to be positive, even in times of depression.

He continued with his fasting and noticed more improvements. He conquered disease and managed to rejuvenate his physical body. Everything but God now seems secondary to him. He is full of gratitude and says that he never felt better in his whole life, not even when he lived with his wife and children, when he had a home and his profession as an architect. He is convinced that God never abandons anybody, only that He lovingly guides us to fulfill our destiny.

He has become an example to his fellow prisoners. Despite his physical confinement, there is a joy beyond description in him. He is full of gratitude for the awakening that has happened to him. He sees the hard work in the fields as an opportunity to exercise his body, his confinement as a blessing to meditate, and to contemplate his relationship with God. To him, the days of fasting are an opportunity for his purification, and he sees the simple meals of rice and beans as a gift that contributes to his wellbeing. Without being aware of it, it seems that he gradually became a saint. Through his own effort, mainly through fasting, he took the opportunity to transform himself.

Many of us live in freedom and complain about the weather, interest rates, the behavior of others, gasoline prices, and other things. We suffer, because we do not agree with what is happening, and yet, we all have a choice to either accept things or do the best we can to change them. To me, my friend in prison is an example in the way he deals with his situation. Despite of his limited resources and his confinement, he is so full of joy, grateful that God is showing him a way to come Home.

Diet and the Scriptures

Most people use their early years to make money, sometimes at the expense of their health. Later on, they use the money to get their health back. The second part of our life can be the most important one. We have gained more wisdom and in many cases the ability to pursue our most important goals. Probably we formed a family, own our own home, and gained professional experience. It can be a wonderful time for a number of enterprises, provided our health allows it. We could start a new hobby, travel, study, or pursue other interests. The key is to remain healthy to do so. There are many opportunities to acquire more knowledge on the subject and some timeless advice can even be found in the Scriptures.

Those suggestions are just as valid today as they were thousands of years ago. Our body was designed in such a wonderful way that it cleanses and heals itself continuously, unless we waited too long and came to a point of no return. God wants us to be healthy. Wellness is not a matter of money or intelligence. Neither is it a secret revealed to only a few chosen ones. As long as we follow the laws of Nature we can remain healthy, although leading a simple life in a demanding environment may not always be easy.

Even if we decide to rely on the skills of medical professionals and health care practitioners, we still have to do our part. A perfect example of the most natural lifestyle would be animals in the wild. They remain in excellent condition until their last days. There is such grace, such beauty, such perfection in them as we hardly find it in human beings. Animals know what to eat, when to eat, they exercise, and they have none of the ailments we find in humans. Baldness, pimples, rotten teeth, varicose veins, shortness of breath, poor eyesight, weight problems, or stiffness of joints are unknown to them. They keep their teeth, their colors, their shape, their eyesight, hearing, and agility almost to the end. They always know what is best for them. We humans were created perfect as well, but often we forget what is best for us, especially when it comes to food and we like to overeat.

Animals keep their food intake simple. Some species like to eat grass and leaves, others fruit or grains, and others are meat eaters. They drink water, and once they satisfy their appetite, they stop eating. When animals are sick, they fast until their health returns. It is possible to survive long periods of time without food. Polar bears, for example, hibernate about six months and in spring they look just as cuddly and strong as they did before. Humans panic at the thought of not eating for a day. Some get irritated when they don't have their coffee in the morning. Actually, it is surprising how much abuse the body can take before it starts to react in a negative way.

In a way, animals can be our teachers or we can learn from others. We also have the Scriptures to provide us with guidelines for a long and healthy life. We are children of the most High, and He surely wants us to have a good life, so we can praise Him in gratitude.

In the Bible*, we find specific indications on food in Genesis 1:29. It says: "I have given you every herb yielding seed, which is upon the face of all the earth, and every tree which bears fruit yielding seed. To you it shall be for food." This passage recommends a diet consisting of fruit, vegetables, grains, seeds and herbs as the most adequate one. It is a diet that even in modern times is recommended as one of the most health promoting ones. The Greek physician Hippocrates (460-372 BC) also stressed the importance of natural food for health in his famous words: "May thy food be thy medicine and thy medicine thy only food." Up to this day, medical doctors still swear the Oath of Hippocrates, which recommends first of all to do no harm. Well intentioned as doctors may be, many of their procedures have side effects and harmful consequences. Hippocrates recommended a diet void of any food which would not fall under the category of "medicine" or improve our wellbeing.

Yogis study the teachings of the Vedas, the Holy Scriptures of the Hindus. Many of them remain youthful to an advanced age. Although yoga positions are health promoting, the main goal of all yoga practices is to extend our life span and serve God as long as possible. Yogis consider their body the temple of God and give it the best possible care through diet, fasting, breathing exercises, certain postures, and meditation. The result is that some of them look as if they were in their thirties when their real age is beyond 100.

The Vedas originated over 5,000 years old, and their wisdom is part of other religions as well. Food was classified into three categories: sattvic, rajasic and tamasic. Sattvic means superior or excellent and consists of foods which maintain the body strong and healthy, promoting longevity, intelligence, happiness and joy. It is a diet that consists mainly of fruit, vegetables, milk, (probably raw milk), butter, nuts and grains. Such foods are highly recommended for people who wish to follow the path of yoga (union with God) or for anybody who wishes to attain a superior state of health.

Rajasic, i.e. of medium quality or stimulating foods, include those that are bitter, acid, salty, very hot, pungent, dry or burning. It is the kind of food that has been cooked with a lot of spices and is very tempting to the taste buds. Here we find meat, fish, eggs, alcohol and similar substances. A rajasic diet increases animal passion and in the long run causes disturbances in our nervous and circulatory system. Today's so-called balanced diet is a rajasic diet.

The third kind of food is tamasic, inferior or impure, and it consists of food which is only half cooked, tasteless, rotten, spoiled, overripe or dirty. Such food makes a person awkward and lazy.

Foods from the highest category in combination with exercise, occasional fasting, the application of water, earth, light, massages, the use of gems, sound, fragrances and colors are also practiced under the name of Ayurveda, the Science of Life. It is an ancient art of healing through purification, which ultimately leads to rejuvenation. Apart from a vegetarian diet, yogis keep a few other guidelines. They recommend to:

*   not overeat and chew food well, especially starches;
*   ingest food at room temperature, neither very hot nor very cold. Both are harmful to the digestive tract;
*   occasionally fast for internal purification and when under stress, since in those times the body does not produce enough hormones and enzymes for digestion.
*   The process of cooking, canning and preserving destroys vitamins, enzymes, and other vital ingredients. Chemical additives, hormones, pesticides and antibiotics fall in the same category and should be avoided.
*   They suggest not to smoke, since each cigarette neutralizes approximately 23 milligrams of vitamin C,
*   and to avoid alcohol, because it has a harmful effect on our glandular and nervous systems.

There is always some good in every situation. Perhaps, sometimes there is a lesson to be learned and we don't see it right away, but we can ask for help. God might then send us His angels in human or invisible form. Maybe the answer comes through a thought, a book, a person or in some other unexpected way. I used to think that God speaks our language, and that He only speaks to selected persons, especially when one of the pastors repeatedly affirmed that last night God spoke to him. I did not hear anything. Apparently, I had the wrong expectations. He speaks to all of us, although often not audibly to our physical ears. The answer to our prayers may come as a thought, a dream, an idea or as an event or circumstance.

The Bible* gives us guidance for many situations in our life. Diet is no exception. The best-known story on diet can be found in the Book of Daniel 1, verse 3-20. It says that Nebuchadnezzar, the King of Babylon, had chosen a few young men in whom there was no blemish, who were handsome in their appearance and skillful in all wisdom, to teach them the learning and language of the Chaldeans. The king appointed for them a daily provision of his delicacies and of the wine which he drank, and three years of training. Among these young men were Daniel and three of his friends. Daniel decided in his heart that he would not defile himself and eat of the King's delicacies nor drink of the wine which he drank. He requested of the chief of the eunuchs that he would not force him to eat.

The chief of the eunuchs was afraid that if the faces of Daniel and his friends looked worse than those of the other boys, the king would have him beheaded. But Daniel pleaded with him: "Test your servants for ten days and give us vegetables to eat and water to drink. Then let our appearance and the appearance of the boys who eat of the king's delicacies be examined, and as you see, deal with your servants." So the head of the eunuchs consented and tested them for ten days. At the end of the ten days he saw that their countenances were much fairer and fatter than those of all the boys who ate of the king's delicacies. Thus, he took away the portion of their food and the wine that they should drink and gave them "pulse" (vegetables) to eat and water to drink.

When the days that the king had commanded were over, the chief of the eunuchs brought them in before King

Nebuchadnezzar. And the king found none among all of them like Daniel and his friends. In all matters of wisdom and understanding that the king inquired of them he also found them ten times better than all the magicians and astrologers in his whole realm.

In the case of Daniel and his friends, we see that a vegan diet, apart from promoting health and physical beauty, is also capable to produce clarity of mind and superior intelligence.

Regardless of whether we choose to eat meat, vegetables, or both, our food should be as natural as possible, without much processing and harmful additives. It is only when we deviate from the Divine laws that we become ill. We tend to blame our problems on a malicious microbe or other outward sources and expect our physician to help us with pills, injections, or surgery. We created the problem and it is up to us to take responsibility and make changes for the better.

The original diet recommended for man was vegetarian, although such a diet was never popular with the masses. The Judeo-Christian tradition, as well as other religions, eventually allowed certain types of meat. Muslims eat fruit, vegetables, grains, fish and some meat. Pork and alcohol are still forbidden.

Mazdaznan, an ideology which originated in Persia before the conversion to Islam and was founded by Zoroaster, also stresses the importance of a vegetarian diet. One of its followers, Dr. Otoman Zar'Adusht Ha'nish (1844-1936), not only lived on a strict vegetarian diet, but also fasted many times for forty days or longer. At the age of sixty, he looked no older than twenty-five. His features were well defined, like those of a young man. In a later photograph taken in Berlin, Germany, in 1932, Dr. O'Hanish looked like a man in his seventies standing straight and tall. Some believe that he was born in 1820, which would have made him over one hundred years old at the time.

In our time, we are used to eating meat, although some people follow a vegetarian diet with excellent results. Others thrive on meat or a mixed diet. In fact, some of the longest living people include some meat or fish in their diets. Jesus himself was not vegetarian. Although it seems that He did not eat every day and fasted for forty days, He ate fish and drank wine. The emphasis seems to be on the amount of food and frequency with which we eat.

Eating less has always led to superior health, mainly in combination with exercise or outdoor work. Poor people tend to enjoy better health because by nature they have to walk more and sometimes cannot afford more than one simple meal a day. The decisive factor seems to be what else we consume in addition to vegetables, meat, or both.

Anything we put in our system has its consequences. Although food is important, other things count as well. How often do we eat and at what times? What kind of medication do we take? Do we exercise? What about the quality of the air and water in our environment? What are our family values?

To achieve a sense of wellbeing, we also need inner peace. Although our food should be as simple and natural as possible, we also have other needs. There is exercise, even if it is just walking outdoors for a few minutes every day. A good diet is only part of our well-being. To be healthy, we also need to be at peace with ourselves, to be honest in our dealings with others, and maybe read the Scriptures for guidance and inspiration.

Greens and Minerals for Life!

Minerals are electrolytes, and since our body is basically electromagnetic energy, they are vitally important to make everything function well. What we call food is a combination of vitamins, minerals, protein, carbohydrates, fats, and water. In raw foods, we also find enzymes and receive the additional benefit of color and fragrance.

Green is the most predominant color in nature, and green leafy vegetables and grasses are probably the most perfect food we can find. Animals can live on grass and leaves, why shouldn't we be able to live on them as humans? It is important to include one salad or green smoothie every day in our diet in order to stay healthy because greens include most of the required minerals, some vitamins, and fiber, all in the right combination.

Minerals are so important because they are involved in just about every function of the body. Most nutritionists believe they need to be organic to be of maximum benefits. Whereas plants can absorb inorganic minerals from the soil and convert them into organic ones, humans and animals have to go through plants or animals for absorption.

Absorption is the key because it is not what we ingest that counts, but rather the degree to which the nutrients are being absorbed. Deficiencies, often caused by the intake of refined sugar, may be the cause of multiple disturbances. Deficiencies can also be caused by parasites or fungus, remaining undetected for years. Parasites feast on vitamins and minerals, and it is of utmost importance to get rid of them first. Once parasites are in the body, some of them reproduce quickly, laying thousands of eggs a day. Fungi are even more dangerous. They are capable of suffocating healthy cells and organs. An overgrowth of a fungus like Candida is the cause of many degenerative and some so-called killer diseases. It is important to keep our immune system strong, mainly through organic minerals, and we find them particularly in green leafy vegetables.

Minerals are necessary to repair damaged tissues. Professor Linus Pauling (1901-1998) was awarded the Nobel Prize in chemistry in 1954. He claimed that **all disease is due to mineral deficiencies**. How is it possible that Americans in one of the wealthiest nations of the world and with food being more than plentiful, suffer from deficiencies? The answer is simple: the average person consumes a lot of empty calories with few or no minerals. Junk food may look and taste like real food, but it has hardly any nutrients in it.

Many companies add chemicals to their "food" to make it look appetizing, trying at the same time to save money. Instead of real juice, we may get colored water with gas, harmful sweeteners, and artificial flavor. A package of strawberry and cream packaged gelatin may look very appetizing, but among the ingredients inside the box you will neither find cream nor strawberries. Even bread can feel like soft cotton with all the original nutrients removed.

One of my clients used to work in a bread factory in Mexico. I mentioned to him that I had been trying to bake my own bread with whole grains, but that the dough did not rise and the bread was hard like rock afterwards. When I asked about a better way, assuming he would know, he said that in the factory where he worked he had never seen flour or grains. He said that they poured a liquid with certain chemicals into the forms and that he had no idea what was in them, definitely not whole grains. Nowadays, consumers are becoming more aware and read the labels with the ingredients, whether it applies to bread or any other food. However, due to their economic situation many people still choose the cheapest product.

Premature aging, tiredness, poor memory, negative mental states, and several previously unknown diseases may all be due to a lack of minerals, which either are not present in our food or which the body is unable to absorb. As our soils have become more depleted, our food has become less nutritious. An ever-increasing number of ailments shows up with no cure in sight. For a cure, we need to look to nutrition, not to surgery and chemicals. Our immune system can only rebuild itself from the inside out. If we ate organic, unprocessed food, free from pesticides, growth hormones and other additives, our weight problems, dental caries, depression, lupus, psoriasis, skin diseases and almost everything else would be non-existent or could be quickly reversed.

It may take years before mineral deficiencies are detected. We think it is normal to gain more weight or feel tired, or that dental problems start showing up due to our age. The change is so gradual and without pain that we tend to believe we are healthy. A lack of minerals affects our bones, hair, teeth, weight, skin, heart, brain, reproductive system and energy levels. It can influence the functioning of each and every organ. We depend on minerals for health and beauty. Minerals make the difference between lasting youthfulness and premature aging.

Minerals affect our hormones, digestion, energy, enzyme production, even our state of mind and our emotions. A lack of certain minerals may cause depression, apathy, even a desire to commit suicide. A weight problem may not be due to overeating as it is widely assumed, but may well be due to a lack of iodine causing thyroid malfunctioning. Heavy people often eat very little in fear that they might gain even more weight, whereas the skinny ones tend to eat a lot trying to gain weight. In either case, their metabolism is not working properly.

There are approximately 120 minerals and trace minerals known to influence our well-being. Some of them can be synthesized by the body. Others, the essential ones, need to come from the outside. A lack of any one of them over time may cause serious disturbances. Trace minerals are only required in small amounts, but are equally important. If any one is missing over a prolonged period of time, deficiencies and malfunctioning are the result. Planet earth and the oceans contain all necessary minerals but we cannot eat soil and rocks. The body only absorbs minerals in their organic state. We need to consume plants, meat, or fish. Thus, the minerals have been converted into organic ones and come in the right combination with other minerals, fats, vitamins, water, and protein

Following is a chart as an example, which shows how the mineral content in food has decreased over the years, especially after chemical fertilizers were used to accelerate the growth of crops. The iron contents in a medium-sized raw apple with skin declined by an unbelievable 96.09 % between 1914 and 1992. It is not likely that things have improved much afterwards.

Mineral contents of an apple:

	1914	1963	1992	Change
Calcium	13.5 mg	7.0 mg	7.0 mg	- 48.15 %
Phosphorous	45.2 mg	10.0 mg	7.0 mg	- 84.51 %
Iron	4.6 mg	0.3 mg	0.18 mg	- 96.09 %
Potassium	117.0 mg	110.0 mg	115.0 mg	- 1.71 %
Magnesium	28.9 mg	8.0 mg	5.0 mg	- 82.70 %

The biggest drop occurred between 1914 and 1963, the years when chemical fertilizers were introduced. Around the turn of the century, about 85 percent of the population in the

United States used to live on farms and grew their own food. Part of the crops were returned to the soil to ensure minimal depletion. Today, as the population has grown and more people live in cities with an ever-increasing demand for food, farmers try to raise several crops a year by using chemical fertilizers.

The result is bigger and prettier fruits and vegetables with less taste and fragrance and fewer nutrients. Genetically modified foods are even more harmful. The only way to avoid them is to pay a higher price for organic produce. Some of us may still remember the times when strawberries tasted and smelled like strawberries and apples gave off a delicious fragrance during the winter months. Today, we have to pay extra to get at least some of the vital nutrients by buying organically grown produce.

Recently, the ingestion of small amounts of purified ocean water has been rediscovered in some countries as a panacea for disease. The reason is that ocean water has each mineral and trace mineral known to man. It contains all 118 elements of the periodic table. A word of caution: since ocean water is salty, even in small amounts and diluted to simulate the amount of salt present in our blood, people who suffer from high blood pressure need to monitor themselves. Ocean water contains magnesium and should not affect blood pressure, but to be on the safe side, observe your reaction if you decide to ingest it. Usually a teaspoon or a tablespoon a day diluted in spring water is sufficient. Purified ocean water is easily available in Europe.

In countries like Germany, France, and Spain it has been used for years. It is also sold in Mexico and South America, especially in Nicaragua, where it has been applied with great success in clinical environments. It is consumed by ordinary people for its mineral contents and wonderful health benefits.

Since minerals are so important, I would like to mention a few of them and also where you can find them.

Calcium intervenes in many bodily functions like bone building, the nervous system, hormone regulation, etc. It is destroyed at temperatures above 150 degrees Fahrenheit or with the consumption of coffee or refined sugar. We find it in blue-green algae, green, leafy vegetables, nuts, seeds, fresh egg yolk, fish, cabbage, onion, and whole grain bread among others.

Iron is necessary for the absorption of oxygen. Without iron, we are unable to use oxygen, and without oxygen we cannot live. A lack of iron and calcium may be the cause of fibroid tumors, which over a third of women in the U.S. suffer from. Green, leafy vegetables and blackstrap molasses contain both iron and calcium, and have been reported to reverse fibroid tumors in some cases. Inorganic iron weakens the kidneys, and experiments with rats showed that giving them inorganic iron caused their death in less than thirty-three days. Good sources of organic iron are all greens, as well as black cherries and their juice.

Without **magnesium,** life on earth would be impossible. Chronic constipation frequently is due to a lack of magnesium. Its lack may also be the cause of impotence. We find it in all yellow and green fruits and vegetables. Its absorption is reduced when ingesting coffee, candies, alcohol, cigarettes, or bread baked with yeast.

A deficiency in **iodine** may cause nervousness, flabby skin, irritability, heart and lung problems, weight gain and hair loss. We find it in fish and all seafood, blue-green algae, eggs, sea vegetables, and fruits that grow close to the ocean. Our body is also capable of absorbing iodine through the soles of our feet. A walk along the beach or a foot bath with unrefined sea salt can be beneficial in activating our entire metabolism.

Chlorine is considered a great blood purifier. It has to be organic though. In its inorganic form, as we find it in many household cleaners, it can be lethal. If you use it for cleaning, the room needs to be ventilated as soon as possible afterwards.

Sodium maintains our joint flexibility and gives our body a youthful appearance. Its lack may cause infertility. White table salt has the opposite effect. It is not compatible with the human body! A lack of organic sodium may cause infertility.

Years ago, German engineers were sent to help with the construction of a steel plant in Rourkela, India. Apparently, they were not used to the hot climate where people sweat a lot and lose sodium. Their wives, who went with them, were unable to conceive until they were given an additional ration of sodium, mainly in homeopathic form, and the problem subsided. We find organic sodium in beef broth, sour milk, celery, fish, apples, and lentils among others.

Potassium balances sodium. Both minerals in their organic form make our blood more alkaline, less prone to disease. Potassium promotes hair growth, is necessary for proper functioning of the heart muscle, and improves rheumatic and arthritic conditions. Its lack may cause water retention, lack of ambition, isolation, and restlessness. A good source of potassium is brown rice, as well as almonds, watercress, and goats' milk.

Silice is another mineral which nearly everybody has not enough of and, like organic sodium, is considered a youth mineral. High amounts can be found in diatomaceous earth and oats. Due to its contents of silice, regular consumption of oatmeal can do more for hair, skin, and fingernails than most beauty products.

A diet rich in **Sulfur** guarantees beauty and youthfulness. People who are low in sulfur may suffer from psoriasis, skin diseases, scalp infections, hair loss, baggy eyes, a continuous desire for food, and an inability to get up in the morning. An organic form called MSM, or Methylsulfonylmethane, is available in health food stores. Among other benefits it improves hair growth.

Oxygen is particularly important because in every case of heart problems this is the principal element lacking.

Foods containing iron, like leafy green vegetables, help in the absorption of oxygen. Larger quantities are in the air we breathe. Therefore, exercise is so valuable. It also makes our skin rosier, which makes us more attractive to the opposite sex.

All minerals and trace minerals are important and they need to be organic. Any time we do not feel or look our best we can be sure that minerals are missing. Which ones? It is hard to determine. It could be any of the trace minerals we have not even heard of like beryllium, cesium, gadolinium, neodymium, or thorium. Whether we know about them or not, our body needs them. Researchers have come up with proof that minerals like cesium or germanium are lacking in cancer patients.

In the United States, the lack of minerals is so rampant that we **must** use adequate supplements. Nutrient rich, organically grown foods, healthy oils, and adequate protein on a daily basis are more needed than ever to stay young. Our best choice may be to eat a variety of wholesome foods, especially greens in salads or green smoothies, some fruit, nuts, grains, and small amounts of cold unprocessed oils. Meat, eggs, and fish might not be as bad as their reputation is among vegetarians. They should, however, be organic whenever possible and only be consumed in small amounts. Processed and packaged foods with artificial additives are probably much more harmful than a piece of meat.

A good way to get most of the required nutrients into our body in the right amounts and right combinations may be through supplementation, especially with green foods. Chlorella, Spirulina, barley, alfalfa, and greens in general are helpful and may increase our wellbeing and beauty. There are reports that people in their seventies managed to restore their own hair color. Others have reversed disease. To include mineral rich food is vital at any age to maintain and restore good health. Cravings and inexplicable aches and pains will disappear as well.

Raw green leafy vegetables and certain organically grown supplements are full of valuable nutrients. A salad a day might certainly keep the doctor away, and a green smoothie or fresh juice with all its organic minerals is absorbed even faster. Many years ago, I came across another strong believer in the power of green juices. His name was Karl Duda and he used to teach in vegetarian restaurants in Mexico City. He was in his late seventies and had just gotten married to a beautiful Mexican lady in her thirties. He was tall and slim, and danced and sang until late in the evening, accompanying himself on the piano. He always invited his students to join him in his joyful enterprise and sometimes it was hard for us to keep up with him. On one occasion, he related the story of his aunt Margarita in Germany. This lady had had a mastectomy at the age of fifty-two due to breast cancer and was told by several eminent physicians that she would not last more than a year. Her father and her uncle, both medical doctors, desperately tried to save her. However, they all came to the same sad conclusion that she could not last more than a year. Her nephew, Karl Duda, advised her to live exclusively on raw spinach juice for a month. She was skeptic, but not having too many other options, she eventually agreed to give it a try. In those thirty days, she lost about fifty pounds and the cancer was gone by the end of the month. She lived for many more years in good health and only died forty years later, at the age of ninety-two, and to everyone's surprise without ever suffering from another disease.

There is no need for drastic fasting unless you want to turn your health around without further delay. One green smoothie a day is sufficient. Even if you eat other foods as well, soon you will notice the effects on your skin, hair, and fingernails. You will experience more energy and lose weight. A smoothie can be made by blending leafy green vegetables like spinach, kale, parsley, and cilantro. Also, celery, cucumber, or carrot tops can be used, adding some fruit to improve the taste. You might want to add barley grass, alfalfa, or blue green algae in powder form for extra chlorophyll.

One of my favorites is moringa, a recently discovered miracle food from a tree which originates in India and also grows in some parts of Africa. Chia and hemp seeds are not green, but they add valuable nutrients to the mixture. Consuming a green smoothie over time is probably the most powerful beauty drink you can come up with. It might improve your complexion and rejuvenate your whole body. Hair and skin will look different and you can't even imagine what it does to your energy. Some people prefer to juice their greens instead of blending them. This removes the fiber, but the nutrients are better absorbed by the body and it gives excellent results. Bear in mind that adding different ingredients might be healthier, but it will also make the smoothie less palatable when it gets too thick. It is best to keep it simple.

A client of mine is another living testimonial of the power of green drinks. When I first met her, she had just had a hysterectomy. She was overweight, felt depressed, her hair and eyes were without luster, and she looked swollen and bloated. She used to be busy taking care of her kids and her ailing father. Her husband was an ordained minister and she helped him at the church. She said that lately she had not found the strength to move about as usual. I asked her if she was willing to try a green smoothie for a month, even if it did not taste too good. She agreed and did not come back the following month. In the meantime, she sent me referrals and they all told me how wonderful she looked. I thought these people must be exaggerating because this was not how I remembered her and did not pay much attention to their reports.

After about six months, she finally came back to see me and I could hardly believe my eyes. She looked years younger, like a different person. She was slim now, her eyes sparkled and her hair looked very shiny and she had a big smile on her face. What a transformation! Like coming out of a cocoon and changing into a beautiful butterfly. She looked radiant and seemed to have found a new desire for life. She had been drinking the green juice almost every day and said that her husband was drinking it too, and that it had helped them both in coping with their busy schedules.

The green drink is one of the most powerful tools for a fast recuperation in any kind of health challenge. Not only is it healing, it helps eliminate putrid matter from the body, it supplies the blood stream with vitamins A, D, and E and important minerals like calcium, magnesium, and iron. It also contains fiber, enzymes, and fresh chlorophyll. The parsley added to the spinach rids the body of excess water and may help to improve eyesight.

Ann Wigmore, who was famous for promoting sprouts and wheatgrass juice for health, experienced such tremendous changes in her own body that she opened a health center in the U.S. In one of her books, she reports that apart from curing her arthritis and other ailments, even being in her late seventies, her gray hair took its natural color again and stayed that way until the day she died, which was in a fire in 1993.

Green juices and smoothies may benefit each one of us. Another advantage is they can also be consumed by people who do not like salads and for whom it is easier to drink their greens.

The results are always startling.

Our Own Fountain of Youth

If there was one thing that could help you return to health, look younger, increase your level of energy, has no side effects, and does not cost you a penny, would you go for it?

Most people would get suspicious and answer something like "it depends." Others would perhaps shrug it off as too good to be true. There is such a remedy accessible to all of us. It is our own urine, also called our own perfect medicine because it contains hundreds of elements like vitamins, minerals, hormones, enzymes, protein, and other substances yet to be analyzed. The body manufactures this concoction every day, different for each one of us according to our specific needs. Urine as a therapy has been used with great success for all kinds of ailments internally and externally for many, many years. Its main ingredient, urea, has also been used in medicines and some beauty preparations. Since it is considered a waste product, people may shudder at the idea of ingesting it unless they are highly motivated and try it to alleviate an otherwise incurable condition. Nevertheless, there are thousands of testimonials about the miraculous effects of urine therapy.

In Hindi scriptures, it is mentioned as "Shivambu," the nectar of God. Others call it the "water of life" or "your own perfect medicine." Most people are reluctant to drink their own pee because it is considered toxic, and also, even if it did help them, it does not make them more attractive to talk about it. A gentleman who healed himself of an incurable disease was so enthusiastic about it that he wanted to convince everybody about this miraculous liquid. After a while even his own family was afraid to invite him for dinner because he talked about nothing else.

At one time, I had my own radio show in Mexico on natural medicine and people used to call in. The idea of drinking urine was quite foreign to me and when a woman called in to ask for my opinion I had to give her an answer on the air. Not wanting to appear totally ignorant about the subject I told her that it had been used for centuries (I had heard that much about it) and if it worked for her to go ahead and drink it. I did not want to tell her what I really thought about the therapy and about people who drink pee. Besides, no negative side effects had ever been reported, so I thought it was okay to encourage her with her practices.

A week later she made an appointment to see me for a diet, and to my surprise she was not some crazy old pervert, but a gorgeous looking young woman in her twenties. Her eyes were sparkling and so clear as I had only seen them in young children. Her skin was soft like velvet. She had a beautiful mane of shiny black hair. She, her husband, and a friend of hers, who was pregnant, all claimed that they had been on urine therapy for over a year and that they all felt great. All three of them seemed indeed to be in the best of health. They had a great sense of humor and were used to laughing at the jokes others made at their expense. It did not seem to bother them a bit.

A few weeks later I heard another miracle story from a dear friend of mine. She was taking care of a man in his late eighties who was bedridden due to advanced prostate cancer. The old man had been given up on by the doctors. He looked pale, emaciated, and lay in his bed, ready to die. He had little appetite and my friend Maria, who was in her seventies herself, was hired by the family to take care of him for as long as he was breathing, which they expected to be not more than a few months at the most. Maria was happy and grateful for the extra income.

The family had hired her despite her own advanced age and poor health. One afternoon, Maria had the television running and the program caught her attention. It was Christina Salghieri's show from Florida. She called the old man and they both watched with fascination. The program showed people from all walks of life giving their testimonials about what drinking their own urine had done for them. Some claimed this therapy had healed them from ulcers, cancer, arthritis, allergies, high blood pressure, hair loss, and so much more. It seemed like a miracle therapy. Drinking urine had been the answer for them, often as a last resort, and it cost nothing.

The old man did not have much to lose. The doctors had given him up and his cancer was not getting any better. He decided to give it a try. After about three months he seemed fully recovered. He gained weight and his skin color returned to a rosy pink. Maria, his caretaker, then decided to give it a try too and became a regular pee drinker herself.

In about a year's time, they both looked rosy, well-nourished and full of energy. Maria claimed that her allergies were gone, and so were the age spots on her hands and the wrinkles on her face. She mentioned that while she had been flat-chested all her life, she now was not so skinny anymore and her body had acquired some new curves she never had before. Then, one day, the old man fell and broke his hip. He had to go to the hospital and Maria was distressed. Being close to ninety, a recovery seemed highly unlikely for him, and her client would probably not make it out of the hospital, which meant that she would be without a job. Remembering his success in the past, the man started drinking his urine in the hospital as soon as he felt a little better. He was released, and after another month to everybody's amazement he drove his truck again and the family rehired Maria to look after him.

There are hundreds, or maybe even thousands, of people from all over the world who have successfully tried this therapy, often in combination with a healthier diet, like Amber, whom I mentioned earlier, and who lived a month exclusively on fruit and juices. She combined her diet with urine therapy, and experienced tremendous changes in her appearance and the way she felt. People report that skin conditions clear up, allergies disappear, blood pressure goes back to normal, hair growth improves, athletes foot gets healed, excessive pounds melt away, and on and on. Although the therapy is at least 5,000 years old, modern scientists are aware of the benefits and have incorporated urea, its main ingredient, in many costly beauty preparations and medicines. Under these circumstances, if inclined to do so, one might choose to apply one's own urine instead of paying for somebody else's.

Another believer is my friend Jacob. Although he is a wealthy man, he remains humble and open to new ideas. Whenever his business allows him to take time off, he goes for a few days to a health center and combines the supervised fasting programs with his self-imposed urine therapy. He looks fabulous. He also learned about the therapy by accident. His sister-in-law used to work at a bank in Mexico. She and the manager had embezzled a large amount of money and fled to the U.S. to escape prosecution. First, they went to Las Vegas and gambled, hoping to make more money. Instead, they lost it all and both, now penniless, had to live in their car. Apparently, with the police after them and having had to leave her own country practically overnight, the young woman had a lot of stress. Her hair fell out in patches and a huge tumor formed on her head. Without money and nowhere to go, she asked Jacob if she could stay at his house until she found a way to make a living. He agreed to let her stay there. The tumor was growing and she could not go back across the border because the police was looking for her. She begged Jacob to take her to a hospital to see what could be done. The doctors advised surgery, which would cost about $80,000. She did not have the money for the operation. By coincidence, she found two books on urine therapy and started reading them. The stories were fascinating to her, and not having anything to lose, she decided to give it a try and started drinking urine without telling anybody and rubbing some on her head.

After about three to four months when Jacob saw that her tumor had practically disappeared and her hair had grown back, thick and beautiful like before, he asked her what she had been doing. She then told him that she had been drinking her own urine every day. She commented that the taste was okay, only when she ate fish the taste got bad. Jacob said he would never have believed it if he had not seen the changes with his own eyes. He now also drinks a glass or so sporadically to keep himself in good shape. He says it is his secret for staying young.

Urine therapy has been used all over the world. It is believed to have originated in India. It is mentioned in the Damar Tantra as part of India's 5,000-year-old holy scriptures, the Vedas. Yogis study these scriptures as part of their training and many of them manage to conserve their youthful appearance to an advanced age. It is hard to tell how much, how often, and when they drink it, whether they use urine therapy in addition to other practices or not, because it is not something they advertise. Most likely, they follow a vegetarian diet, special breathing exercises, meditation, and the practice of certain yoga positions, which all contribute to longevity and a youthful appearance.

The Indian scriptures mention that God Shiva gave his wife Parvati a recommendation to drink urine every day in combination with a light diet. He suggested to drink the middle flow of the first urine in the morning and that this practice is capable of abolishing old age and various types of diseases. Rock salt and raw honey in equal proportions should be taken in the early morning as well. He also warned Parvarti **to not tell anyone.**

Moraj Desai (1896-1995), India's former Prime Minister, was a fervent promoter of urine therapy. He publicly talked about it and believed that it would do wonders to improve the health of the poor in his country. Not only did he drink his own urine, he is said to have had a daily massage with it every morning before taking his bath. Up to his death he had no wrinkles and a full head of hair although he was way over ninety years of age at the time.

In another ancient text, we find that "human urine controls bile in the blood, destroys worms, cleanses the intestines, controls cough and calms the nerves. It is sharp in taste, destroys laziness and is an antidote to poisons."

In her outstanding book *Your Own Perfect Medicine,* Martha M. Christy tells the story of her own healing after thirty years of disease and gives a scientific background with many case histories of this simple therapy. One of the first enthusiastic pee drinkers and therapists was J.W. Armstrong from Britain. In 1945, he published the book *The Water of Life,* which has become a classic, and in which he describes his path from incurable disease to perfect health. He testifies that after a forty-five-day urine fast he lost about 100 pounds and looked fifteen years younger. He also testifies to amazing cures he observed in others through urine therapy after all else had failed and many had been given up by conventional medicine.

Urine can be used internally and externally. If taken internally, it should always be ingested fresh, right after it has been collected, starting out with a few drops collected from the mid-stream and placed under the tongue, and then gradually increasing the amount to an ounce or more twice a day. For external use, the liquid can be a few hours or a day old and even seems to become more effective, especially for skin diseases. Either way, internal or external, there are no known negative side effects.

Urine can be used for a variety of problems, even as a hair tonic when applied to the scalp half an hour before shampooing, or as a mouth wash to improve the health of teeth and gums. Since urine reflects our state of health, its taste in sick people might be nasty and difficult to take in the beginning.

Although I had read and heard a lot about the benefits of drinking one's own urine, I still had my reservations and could not convince myself that this was something I wanted to do. I had also heard that urine was good for plants. I diluted the "elixir" half and half with water and then watered my plants with the mixture. They started growing like crazy, producing wonderful blossoms. My bougainvillea produced beautiful purple colored flowers and the gardenia which was half gone, showed new buttons after a few days. If that is what it can do for plants, there must be some magic ingredients in urine that are also good for humans.

Whether you decide to try urine therapy out of curiosity, to heal yourself of a serious illness, or because you wish to rejuvenate, always remember Shiva's concluding recommendation: "Attempts should be made to keep it a secret. **Do not tell anyone!**"

Is there anything she (or we) would not do to get our quality of life back when all else fails or to look and feel years younger?

It is No Fun to be Acid

Diet does not only affect our physical body. It also affects our personality, our state of mind and general outlook on life. Sourpusses tend to be irritable or depressed, feel lonely and wronged, and there is not much that makes them happy. They tend to complain a lot and hardly ever accept responsibility. Their misery is always somebody else's fault. Sometimes, it seems as if they are just looking for something to complain about. Without being aware of it, such people are acidic, which can be outright dangerous. Due to stress, medications and certain foods they have created an acidic environment with poor health consequently. Fortunately, with a change in diet their state of health and attitude can be reversed.

Our blood should be slightly on the alkaline side, ideally between 7.35 and 7.4. A long-term blood pH under 6.8 or above 7.8 can be deadly. Our blood has to adjust and in order to do so, we need organic alkaline minerals like calcium, magnesium, iron, sodium, manganese, zinc, and potassium. If they are not in our food, the body pulls them from our teeth, bones, and blood vessels. Eating too much protein and refined sugar is not recommended, because they are acid forming. In order to get rid of the acidity the body eliminates alkaline minerals in the process. In an acidic environment, the body cannot absorb oxygen, which can lead to heart problems and other diseases.

Problems seemingly unrelated like excessive hair loss, warts, moles, cancer, kidney stones, hormone imbalances, heart disease, insomnia, caries, cellulite, arthritis, impotency, depression, chronic fatigue, premature aging, and others tend to appear.

There is also a relationship between over-acidity and weight gain, osteoporosis, constipation, fungal overgrowth, low body temperature, infections, loose teeth, brittle nails, infertility, and a deficiency of the immune system. Particularly chronic, degenerative diseases are due to the fact that our blood has been acidic over a long period of time. Parasites, virus, and fungus, they all flourish in an acidic environment, and more often than not happen to be the cause of just about anything that ails us. It is important to restore an alkaline environment because even cancer cells cannot survive in it.

Our blood has been called "a very special juice." It holds the secrets to well-being or disease, to our level of energy, to fast or slow healing, to youthfulness or premature aging, including death. Common blood tests might show the presence of parasites, fungus, virus, elevated blood sugar, triglycerides, or cholesterol, but they hardly ever give a clear picture of our pH values. Our blood will continually try to stay within its normal ranges, trying to balance acidity and alkalinity.

A simple way to find out in what range we are is with a piece of litmus paper. It usually shows pH values between 4.0 and 8.5. The lower numbers indicate higher acidity and the higher ones show a more alkaline state. Values around 7.0 are neutral or ideal. The full scale goes from 1 to 14. It is logarithmic, i.e. a pH (potential of Hydrogen) of 5.0 is ten times more acidic than a potential of Hydrogen of 6.0.

The ideal value lies between 6.8 and 7.4. Urine can be tested at different times of the day although the first morning urine is the most important one. Often, it starts out low around five and then gradually changes to about 7.2 or 7.4 by late afternoon. Some authors consider a morning value of five or 5.5 normal as a result of acid elimination from metabolic activities during the night. Most likely over 90 percent of people find themselves in this range. However, as our diet improves with fruit, vegetables, and herbal teas, the morning urine should also be in the neutral range around seven in a healthy person. Lower values usually indicate a lack of minerals.

In order to be valid, a saliva test needs to be done at least two hours after any food intake. As soon as we eat or drink something, our saliva will change to alkaline. A clever sales lady encouraged prospective clients for her liquid calcium product to test their saliva before and after taking a sip. They started out in the yellow range of the litmus paper, i.e. being too acidic, and were surprised by the rapid change. So they bought the product. Food in general, but especially an alkaline mineral like calcium, instantly changes the saliva and will make the litmus paper green or even dark blue, very alkaline. The question remains: can the body stay in this range? Unless the minerals have been absorbed into the bloodstream, a reading after a sip of an alkaline mineral does not have any validity. It is a sales trick. Repeated checking of your pH at home first thing in the morning will give you a clearer picture, and lets you know whether a change in diet, certain supplements, or a less stressful life have a positive effect on you.

Our body naturally produces acidity because of metabolic processes. We can easily become too "acidic" due to stress, worry, or fear. We can become too acidic due to overeating, intestinal putrefaction, medication, heavy metals, or insufficient chewing. We can become over-acidic by eating too much protein, sugar or carbohydrates. A sedentary lifestyle can likewise cause too much acidity and so can electromagnetic emissions from computers and cell-phones. It is easy to become over-acidic. In nature, acid rain can kill plant life. Fish die in lakes where the pH of the water goes below five. The question is: How can I get back to ideal values within a slightly alkaline range?

Diet is probably the most effective way. A friend of mine owns a pharmacy with her husband. She learned about the importance of alkalizing and applied her newly acquired knowledge to her husband, who was a sick man. She started feeding him more fruits and vegetables, less meat and bread, no refined sugar, and within a few weeks his outlook changed so much that instead of talking about his funeral arrangements they started planning their next vacation.

Sugar is the greatest culprit of all. It feeds yeast and fungus, making us ever more acidic. It also feeds Candida. Consuming refined white sugar is probably one of the fastest ways to acidify our blood. Millions of people suffer from tooth loss, mottled skin, toe nail fungus, insomnia, bone loss and so many other conditions, all attributed to unexplained origins. These problems are difficult to correct because the problem is internal and can only be solved with a strict diet, temporarily avoiding all forms of sugar. If you have an irresistible craving for sweets, and you can be almost sure that it is because of overly acidic blood and an overgrowth of Candida.

In America sugar in some form is added to almost all packaged food. It is added to vegetable soups, canned food, bottled juices, potato chips, baby foods, yogurt (except plain) and just about everything else that is packaged or processed, even fish. According to the Department of Agriculture, it is estimated that Americans now eat about 150 -170 lbs. of sugar a year, whereas it used to be only three to five pounds in the early 1800s.

When we stop ingesting refined sugar, our state of health can be reversed fast. Dr. Mark Stengler from the Institute of Integrative Medicine in Encinitas, California, managed to starve cancer cells to death in some of his patients simply by cutting out all sugar from their diets. Longevity and youthfulness also seem to be in opposite proportion to the amount of sugar we consume.

Consuming refined white sugar is one of the fastest ways to acidify our blood and, therefore, the cause of ailments like diabetes, weight gain, infertility, depression, cancer, allergies, heart disease, arthritis, migraine headaches, mental illness, and many others. George Ohsawa, the founder of macrobiotics, went so far as to say that refined sugar would eventually kill more people in the United States than the atomic bomb. It might be a sweet death, but a death nonetheless. Sugar feeds yeast and fungus, slowly destroying the host.

I learned about the detrimental effects of sugar and the acidity it causes on a visit to Japan. Our tour guide told us that only one generation back few children in Japan wore glasses or had tooth decay. People ate hardly any candy at all. After the country started catering to foreign tourists with sweets, sugared drinks and pastries, and American style fast food restaurants opened, things changed. All these foods cause a high degree of acidity. There have been consequences and nowadays many children use glasses and have to wear braces in their teeth.

Although it is easy to produce acids, either through negative emotions, stress, or the food we eat, the body does not produce alkaline minerals on its own. We must ingest them, especially in the form of green, leafy vegetables. They lead to a more alkaline state, promoting better health and a more positive outlook on life. Acidic fruits do not make our blood more acidic. They trigger chemical reactions which convert over-acidity into neutral values. Sometimes people are afraid to eat citrus fruit or drink lemon juice because they believe that it would only increase their acidity. Just the opposite is true! Fruit acid makes our blood more alkaline. Limes and lemons are among the healthiest fruits available! On the other hand, anything that causes fermentation, like sugar and an excess of protein, increases blood acidity.

Nicolas Capó (1899-1977), a Spanish trophologist, claimed that more than 150 diseases can be cured by daily ingesting the juice of fresh limes or lemons. You can prove it by taking the juice of two limes or lemons daily and notice the difference in the way you feel. After a few days, your pH values will have changed. Although the juice of fresh citrus fruit is acid, it helps the fastest to bring about a neutral pH of around 7.0, thereby eliminating a wide variety of symptoms.

Since the subject of alkalinity and pH values is such an important issue, I would like to mention a few foods that help in alkalizing our blood. These are citrus fruit, especially limes and lemons, melons, green leafy vegetables, sprouts, garlic and onions, asparagus, fresh and powdered barley, wheat grass, chlorella, Spirulina, homemade kefir milk, certain raw oils like extra virgin olive oil, coconut oil, hemp oil, or flaxseed oil, avocados, almonds, herbal teas like chamomile, chaparral, hibiscus, and many others, as well as most vegetables, raw, cooked or juiced.

Acid forming foods to avoid or only to be consumed in small amounts are: meats, bread baked with yeast, pastries, processed foods, cereals, coffee, margarine, canned vegetables, artificial sweeteners, chocolate, white vinegar, chemical additives, and all drugs (prescribed or others).

If your blood has been acidic for a long time, an alkaline diet by itself might not be enough. You will have to take additional supplements and increase your daily intake of leafy green vegetables, drink herbal teas and vegetable juices. Bee pollen, garlic, sprouts or some form of chlorophyll allow for a faster recovery. Pee drinkers should also test their morning urine before they drink it and if the urine stays within the acid range it is recommended to not add insult to injury and wait until the pH goes up to around seven, which might happen later on in the morning or some time during the afternoon. Giving our digestive system a rest or eating only two meals a day instead of three or four, will also greatly improve our health. **Parasites and fungus need to be removed with specific cleanses**. They leach minerals out of the body and keep our blood over-acidic. Parasites leave their waste material behind, which is acidic as well. A colon cleanse, a liver flush and a kidney cleanse with herbs can strengthen our immune system rapidly. So do fasting and almost all mono diets.

A brisk walk outside in the fresh air also raises alkalinity. If you have your litmus paper at hand, measure your saliva or urine before and after the walk. You will notice a change right away. Relaxed vacation time or a walk by the ocean can make a big difference. Ocean water has a neutral value of close to 7.0 pH. During vacation, we tend to stay away from harmful EMFs (electromagnetic frequencies). We worry less, and everything that reduces stress reduces acidity.

Then there is the simple act of chewing. Chewing every bite at least thirty times will raise alkalinity and bring the body back to health. Chewing is probably the most inexpensive and rejuvenating practice of all.

Another aid is an **alkaline bath.** In the past, it has been assumed that healthy skin is supposed to be slightly acidic although a baby's skin is alkaline and so is the water babies are surrounded by when in the womb. Our skin might be mostly acidic because of excretions from inside our body. It might not be its ideal state after all. A very effective way to change the acid/alkaline balance in our favor is by taking a bath in the ocean or in alkaline water. By adding a cup or two of baking soda or Epsom salts to a tubful of warm water, the pH of the water will rise to around 8.5. Remain in the water for at least one hour and make sure the temperature is only around 37 to 38° / 98 to100° F, but does not feel overly hot. When you emerge, and test the bathwater again, you will notice that the pH of the water went down from 8.5 to about 7.5, i.e. your body has given off some of its acid while the acidity of the water has increased tenfold. Conditions like rheumatism, arthritis, night sweats, skin problems and many others are believed to greatly improve with alkaline baths. Also, you might notice your skin has a more pleasant smell and is softer afterwards.

Fungus cannot subsist in a pH above 8.0. In Europe, tubby baths with warm water and alkaline soap once a week used to be common in every household until the bathtub was replaced by the more practical shower. However, a weekly alkaline tubby bath with baking soda or Epsom salts may turn into a healing spa, leaving your skin softer, cleaner, and rosier.

Here is a **million-dollar secret:** It is extremely important to get the pH of our blood into the normal range between 6.8 and 7.4 for **all** metabolic functions. One way to do it is by adding a quarter teaspoon of baking soda to each gallon of drinking water and use it throughout the day. Or, for a certain time, add a dash of baking soda twice a day to a glass of lemonade. It is important not to overdo it, since too much baking soda can make your blood too alkaline and have just the opposite effect. In an emergency, or as a one-time remedy, add half a teaspoon to an eight-ounce glass of water and see how you feel. I tried it once in the evening and felt wonderful the whole next day. The remedy will immediately alkalize your system. You might sleep better and temporarily get a euphoric feeling. The remedy should not be used in the long run, though.

Beautiful, the Natural Way

No matter what we do internally, it can help us to be healthier, but every woman also wants to look good on the outside, and men too, of course. Men go to the gym and exercise. Women spend their money on skin care products. A pretty complexion reflects youthfulness.

When men of different ethnicities were asked what they liked most about a woman, they all agreed that a clear complexion in a woman was one of her most attractive features. It is one of the first things others notice. Our face can reflect worries, lack of sleep, hormone imbalances, water retention, stress, liver problems, etc. On the other hand, it can also reflect good health and self-confidence.

Cosmetics have their place in today's world, and fortunately enough, more and more companies include natural ingredients in their products. Cosmetics can make a difference between looking plain or stunning. The idea is to enhance our natural beauty and hide minor flaws and not make us look like movie stars during the day and totally different at night. A healthy look is "in" at any age, and it is very pretty. In fact, in today's competitive world I think it is necessary to use a little help unless you are young and can be without it. A friend of mine was asked by her boyfriend to not use any make-up because he liked her "natural." She stopped using all make-up, even eyeliner, and she looked much less attractive. If a man likes you to look natural, he probably means not to overdo it.

Skin care products should be as pure and natural as possible. Some enthusiasts go so far as to say that if you can't eat it, don't put it on your skin! Creams, bath additives, lotions, make-up, and costly perfumes make us feel good. We feel pampered and luxurious, but unless you are born perfect, our beauty depends a lot on our diet and inner cleanliness. Diet as well as enemas and colonics can help tremendously to improve our complexion. The famous actress May West had an enema with mineral water every day.

Many store-bought cosmetics contain harmful chemicals. Hydroquinone for example, which is used as a bleaching agent and dark spot corrector, is so harmful that it is banned in Europe. Some other ingredients may be cancer causing. With natural ingredients you cannot go wrong, even if the effect is not as dramatic as you see on TV. You might be tempted to buy a product when you see "before" and "after" pictures in commercials.

Are they real? It is difficult to know because a skillful photographer can do miracles. I remember the last time when I had to renew my passport. The initial picture was not very flattering. I did not want to see myself like this for the next ten years, so I asked the photographer if he could correct the bags under my eyes. He did. I then asked him to soften the lines around my mouth a little and make my teeth look prettier. He complied. His final work came out really good, although he said that he had to stop somewhere because the picture was for a passport and still had to resemble me. The photo now looks the way I would like to look. Maybe it is something to aspire to.

Wearing make-up can make such a difference that some models even admit that if you met them in the street without make-up you might not recognize them. They look gorgeous for the photo shots, and the idea is to sell products. They also know that wearing too much make-up might harm their skin and in their private life many of them use very little.

Cleaning our skin every night before we go to bed is essential and occasionally not wearing any make-up also helps improve our complexion. Drinking enough water, consuming healthy oils like extra virgin olive oil or flaxseed oil, taking vitamins, and getting enough sleep will do more for beauty than the best make-up. A woman at the top of one of the largest cosmetic companies publicly admitted that there is no single product on the market that could actually erase wrinkles. A youthful glow comes from within. Sometimes it happens with a change in diet, sometimes with exercise, sometimes as a result of internal cleansing or spiritual awakening. People dedicated to a spiritual life often look radiant and nothing beats the power of being in love.

If you are single, you may try applying petroleum jelly to your face at night for extra moisture. It looks greasy, but the next morning you will wake up with a soft moist complexion. Freshly squeezed orange juice left on overnight also improves skin texture. It feels soothing and clears your skin. Lime or lemon juice has the strongest effect, especially if taken internally as well. To a young woman with severe acne, I recommended that she put diluted lemon juice on her face for a few moments after cleansing her skin at night and then rinse it off. She misunderstood and left the lemon juice on all night. A month later her complexion was without blemishes, and she was glad she did it despite the initial stinging.

Following are a few natural beauty treatments with proven results:

1) **Honey** has been used in skin preparations for centuries. Whether you have discolorations, blemishes, dryness or small scars, it will take care of them. Mix five tablespoons of thick **raw** honey with one tablespoon of water and one

tablespoon of bay rum. Leave the mixture on for fifteen minutes and then rinse it off. For best results, it should be repeated daily for about a month and you will notice the difference.

2) **Clay** is healing. It penetrates deeply through the skin. For beauty purposes, people recommend French green clay. It has some radioactive effect and helps to reduce wrinkles, acne, and small scars.

3) **Yogurt** works like a gentle peeling due to its lactic acid. Fresh Kefir milk with all its nutrients and enzymes is very effective and can be left on all night.

4) **Brewers' Yeast** is rich in B vitamins, several minerals and amino acids. It is also an excellent source of DNA and RNA, the nucleic acids in our cells. Mix about a teaspoonful of dry yeast with water and leave it on for forty-five minutes to an hour. The mask must be completely dry to be effective. Then peel if off. Your skin will look red and tingle for awhile due to the increased circulation and extra nutrition. Then it becomes rosy and will be soft to the touch.

5) **Grated Carrots and Olive Oil.** A woman in her seventies with no wrinkles at all told me she swore by extra virgin olive oil. She uses it with salads, bread, or by itself, taking a spoonful every morning. She said it kept her young from the inside and did wonders for her skin. Occasionally, she applies a facial mask consisting of grated raw carrots with extra virgin olive oil. She looks wonderful, so her recipe must be working.

6) **Raw Potato Mask.** There is something in raw potatoes that is very soothing and bleaching, evening out skin tone. The latest beauty products in Europe contain potato as one of their main ingredients. As a mask, you can grate the raw potato, mix it with a little milk and then leave it on for about twenty minutes before rinsing it off.

7) **Raw Egg White.** This is a classic. Some women believe it removes wrinkles faster than anything else. Lightly beat the white of an egg and then smooth it on your face. Let it dry and then remove with water after about ten minutes.

A fabulous supplement to improve the appearance of any skin within a short time is cod liver oil taken internally. It has plenty of vitamin A and helps with all kinds of problems. A teaspoonful a day not only improves the health of your heart, bones, and eyes, it also gives you a nice rosy glow.

The most youthful complexions can be seen in people of all ages on a raw food diet. Even women in their sixties often do not look older than somewhere between thirty and forty. Diet is the most powerful way to improve our looks, because it changes our state of health from the inside out. A neighbor of my mother's in Germany told me that she had rented a room to a young teacher. After staying with her for a couple of years, he was transferred to a school in a different town. They stayed in contact with phone calls and occasional greeting cards over the holidays.

Several years later he stopped by to pay her a visit. Great was her surprise when the man, who was now in his sixties and retired, seemed not to have aged at all. In fact, she thought he looked younger than when she last saw him, which was twenty or thirty years ago. He still had his same dark blonde hair and was slim and energetic. She asked him what he had been doing. He said that with all the stress at school he got high blood pressure and put on weight. He often felt tired, but kept working until health reasons forced him to take early retirement and he quit his job.

He heard about the benefits of raw food and started chopping his vegetables, juiced a few times a day, and gradually left all cooked food. Eventually, he bought a trailer and was free to travel and stay wherever he pleased. Sometimes he stayed next to a lake, lived close to a town, by the ocean or near the woods. During the colder seasons of the year he traveled South and then came back in Spring. He started feeling better and better. Finally, he became independent of restaurants and hotels, making his dream come true, to travel and get to know different places and cultures.

I wanted to know more and pressured my friend to try and remember more details. Apparently, he had been on this diet for seventeen years before she saw him again. Besides eating raw food, he stressed that exercise was really important, like walking every day or using a trampoline. Apart from eating raw vegetables and some fruit, he consumed a muesli every morning, which he prepared himself. It was a mixture of oats, nuts and raisins. He admitted that whenever he felt he needed a little more protein he either had a can of tuna fish or a baked potato, but this was rarely the case.

Unless you are born perfect, the key to good health and good looks is diet, diet, diet! African black soap is the most gentle, effective cleanser for the skin. It is made from honey, certain oils, black seeds and tree bark. Another excellent product is rose hip oil. It is supposed to eliminate wrinkles, light scars, even out skin tone and give us the dewy look everybody wants. A gentleman who was selling rosehip oil showed a picture of himself after a motor cycle accident, which had left his skin scarred. He claimed that it was the rosehip oil that restored his skin to normal within two years. Just by using these two products, one should see changes within a short time. I got a lot of compliments when I used them, but I still believe that important changes always come from within.

Enemas and Colonics

It is a topic nobody likes to brag about unless it makes them some money. Natural health care is not complete unless we take care of our intestine, which means to keep it as clean as possible. The large intestine, called the colon, can become a breeding ground for bacteria, parasites, and fungus. Over the years, mucus layers build up with heavy metals, food particles and other residues which remain trapped inside. It may cause fermentation and putrefaction and lead to foul smelling gas and many internal disturbances. The colon of an adult can hold up to thirty pounds of fecal matter!

A diet with enzymes, roughage, water and chlorophyll is helpful to make our bowels move, and even then you may be surprised what the colon can hold. Occasional fasting and supplements to strengthen our liver or parasite and Candida cleanses can help a step further in the right direction. Any form of cleansing means that more is coming out of our body than what was going in. Old, hardened stuff should be removed. Enemas and colonics greatly support the process, especially during times of fasting. Without these internal baths, the body might reabsorb some of the toxic matter we are trying to get rid of. Inner cleansing also has noticeable effects on our skin, since our blood will be purer afterwards. It may also help flatten our stomach, and who would not be interested in looking prettier and having a smaller waistline?

Enemas are not a replacement for good bowel movements and should be done after a natural elimination has taken place. An enema may bring forward a load of undesired waste. In the worst case, it can be in the form of black slime, mucus, root-like structures from yeast, parasites, or nasty smelling chemicals. One of my clients was so sick that when he decided to give himself an enema, what came out was black and purple mud, probably chemicals from medication. Sometimes people get scared when they see the nasty stuff coming out. I find it even scarier when the toxic matter stays inside or is being reabsorbed. People then have to suffer the consequences in form of sickness or premature aging.

Colon cleansing is most important during times of fasting. When people go on a prolonged fast, they tend to feel tired and low in energy without enemas and their recovery will take longer. Those who do enemas while fasting tend to experience very little discomfort. In fact, most of them feel good. During a fast, the body is geared towards elimination and any undesired loosened up waste should be removed from the body as soon as possible. Nobody really likes to do enemas because they are uncomfortable, especially for people who are overweight, elderly or sick, and they should not do them on their own.

If you want to give yourself an enema at home try and make it as simple as possible. The proper equipment might be a little plastic bucket specially designed for the purpose, which holds about a quart and a half of water, or a regular rubber enema bag from the drugstore. I prefer the bucket, because it stands easily on the rim of the bathtub and one can see how much water is left. With either one you have control over the flow. You can wait before you allow more water in or you can release it. The water can be warm or cold. If you want to, you can use herbal tea, coffee, or some additives like a teaspoonful of hydrogen peroxide, chlorophyll, lemon juice or a few drops of oregano oil. Purified water without chlorine is sufficient.

As far as temperature goes, warm water is relaxing and more cleansing whereas cool water is stimulating. In the beginning, you may not be able to hold a lot of water. Don't worry, even if you get only a little water in, expel it, and then try again. You may still be surprised to see what comes out when you look in the toilet. Eventually, blockages will be removed and you may be able to hold more water.

Since the idea is to remove as much waste as possible, it may be helpful to stimulate bowel movements by taking a laxative tea the night before. Herbal teas like **Smooth Move** and **Get Regular** are available in most Health Food Stores. Another option is to stir a teaspoonful of Epsom Salts into a glass of water and drink it in the morning. The cleaner the colon, the better the enema water will penetrate and remove old stuff.

Professionally done, this type of intestinal cleansing is called a colonic or colonic irrigation. It is done with a special machine and is much more comfortable. You lie on a bed or massage table while the trained therapist will insert a disposable plastic tube into your rectum, and the machine will use about 45-60 quarts of purified water to rinse your colon several times, usually during a one-hour session. The effects are more profound than when you do it yourself at home.

Colonics can be expensive, depending on the area where you live. At the therapist's office, the water goes from the disposable tubes through a glass tank that looks something like an aquarium and you can watch the waste coming out. You might see live worms, yeast, fungus, slime, and bile. The therapist will help you interpret the scenery, which can be fascinating. After all, it is you who is involved in the process, not somebody else they are talking about. As the water gets cleaner, you will notice a difference in your overall well-being. Sometimes the therapist can even tell what you have been eating and whether what is coming out is recent or old stuff. As you change your diet, older toxic residue will come out or the water gets cleaner. A session with a therapist is a pleasant experience and nothing to be afraid of. After your visit, you might feel lighter and rejuvenated.

Neither colonics nor enemas are a substitute for an improved diet. Toxins form all over again. It would be like cleaning your house once and believing it stays clean from now on. It won't. You have to continually watch your diet, drink plenty of water and make sure that your food contains fiber and natural enzymes. Special supplements will further help to remove the sludge from your small intestine and push it down into the colon. Some people believe that colonics are harmful because the water removes their good intestinal flora together with the waste. As far as I know, only waste comes out. To be on the safe side, it may be a good idea to take probiotics right afterwards. It is always a personal decision. After a colonic, you might feel so good you want to smile all day long.

An excellent example for a combination of a vegan diet with internal cleansing was Victor Earl Irons (1895-1993). In fact, he invented the Colema Board, which is a hybrid between professional colonic irrigations and enemas. It can be used at home and there are no other expenses than the water. Like many other important naturopaths, in his younger years Mr. Irons lived on junk food, cakes, and candy with a weakness for chocolate bars. As a result, he developed a painful arthritic condition of the spine at the age of forty, which crippled him. He was diagnosed as incurable by six medical doctors in Boston. After reading about natural methods, he turned to cleansing, fasting, natural foods and healing without drugs. Within two months, he had no more pain and within fourteen months there were no more signs of his "incurable" disease.

At the age of seventy-two, Victor Irons began a second family. He fathered his last child at the age of eighty, proof of his vitality and vigor. He passed away in 1993 at the age of ninety-eight from complications of a car accident.

What is so remarkable about Victor Irons? First of all, he was living proof that the recommendations of eating fruit and vegetables do work. In addition to his raw food diet he developed a supplement from the juice of cereal grasses like barley, oats, rye, and wheat. He believed these grasses had high nutritional value and contained every nutrient necessary for all mammals to live on. His most important addition to natural health, however, was the emphasis on intestinal cleaning. He believed the best food, and even the best supplements, are ineffective unless the body can absorb them, which is only possible with proper internal hygiene. He recommended the temporary use of bentonite clay, a powerful absorbent of toxic matter, combined with psyllium husks and stressed the importance of colonic irrigations.

The Colema Board he invented can be used in the privacy of your own home, is less expensive than colonics and more effective than enemas. It is still used with great success in conjunction with a vegetarian diet in several naturopathic centers.

Getting Rid of Harmful Substances

Instead of waiting for an opportunity to change our lifestyle altogether, it is best to make small changes and try to keep them up if they work. It is okay to fail and start again. Temptations will always be there, and small steps on a consistent basis lead to success faster than drastic changes carried out only once.

One of the greatest dangers for all of us are heavy metals. We are hardly ever aware of them, although they seem to affect everyone of us. These substances accumulate gradually in our blood vessels and do not cause pain or other symptoms. Just by being out in traffic and breathing the air of exhaust fumes may allow lead and other heavy metals to enter our blood stream. They can gradually clog up our arteries, affect our brain, our breathing, the nervous and glandular systems, and damage in some way just about every organ. Their presence may affect the skin, our eyesight, joints, cause heart failure, and premature aging.

Other sources of heavy metals are amalgam fillings, cooking in aluminum pots, farm raised fish, the use of deodorants, vaccines, certain cosmetics, tooth paste, food additives, X-rays, the water we drink, asbestos, or contaminated air. There are hundreds of harmful substances everywhere nowadays, and they are not only toxic, but extremely difficult to get rid of. The main ones are lead, arsenic, cadmium, aluminum, mercury, and fluoride.

Alternative medicine offers a process called chelation to remove these heavy metals from our arteries. Usually it is practiced in a medical establishment by physicians with the purpose to avoid heart surgery, and in some cases it can save a person's life. The word "chelation" means "grip." The way the process works is by injecting intravenously a product, usually EDTA. It takes several hours to do so and can be quite expensive since it takes five to thirty sessions to get lasting results. The product is eliminated through the urine together with the heavy metals it binds. Chelation may also pull out calcium, magnesium, and other necessary minerals. Therefore, a trained physician will replace them appropriately without side effects.

In an emergency, chelation may be our least invasive choice. In general, it is best to not wait until the danger of having a stroke or a heart attack is imminent. We can remove heavy metals and other toxins from our arteries continually, either by taking an oral chelation product with natural ingredients or by ingesting certain foods. Once the arteries are clear, the person who underwent the process tends to feel more energy, mental clarity, has better eyesight and skin. Varicose veins diminish and sometimes disappear altogether afterwards.

The most effective foods to remove heavy metals and other toxins from the body are all greens, especially chlorella and cilantro, MSM (a naturally occurring sulphur), vitamin C, selenium, fresh fruit, garlic, enzymes and probiotics. Some of them should be consumed every day. Fasting may also be a very effective way to get results. Vegetarian sources of selenium are Brazil nuts, oats, brown rice, sunflower seeds and spinach. Tuna fish, sardines and salmon are also high in selenium. Recommended are fresh fruit, clean water, juices, greens, or to eat nothing at all until about noon. In fact, the no-breakfast plan has helped thousands of people to improve their health.

Starting the first meal of the day around noon seems to best support our three natural metabolic cycles and can result in tremendous benefits over time. In their international bestseller *Fit for Life,* Marilyn and Harvey Diamond go into detail describing our metabolic cycles. The first cycle is between noon and eight p.m. It is the best time to consume our meals, a time for absorption. During the second cycle, i.e. between eight p.m. and four a.m. nutrients are being used for restoration and repair, and the third cycle between four a.m. and noon, is for elimination. Whenever we start eating, elimination stops. Although new food pushes out waste, elimination itself will be interrupted. Therefore, it is recommended to start with a light breakfast, which could include fruit, a green smoothie, juices or just water. All of them support the process of elimination. Drinking water only with a little lemon juice and optional a clove of garlic may be an excellent way to start the day.

Some people are used to a different eating cycle. They get hungry in the morning and prefer something more filling. It could be a bowl of oatmeal, whole grain bread, eggs or some other source of protein. Especially during the colder seasons of the year, some of us might prefer something warm with more calories. Nothing is written in stone. A bowl of oatmeal with its fiber and B Vitamins is not only tasty, it also benefits our nervous system and hair growth. Since it is best to eat only two meals a day, an option may be to eliminate dinner instead of breakfast.

Greens are among the best chelators we can find, whether they come in form of a salad, a smoothie or juiced. Greens should be consumed at least once a day. They make our blood alkaline and contain almost all nutrients the body needs. Some of the largest animals like the ox, the elephant and the giraffe live on them all their lives. A man by the name of Toro Mattsui near Lake Hakone in Japan lived exclusively on Spirulina for fifteen years. Apparently, it is a complete food and there is no cell or organ in our body that does not benefit from greens. They neutralize acids in our blood. Instead of blending fresh greens, one can mix the powders of Spirulina, alfalfa, chlorella, or barley grass into a glass of freshly squeezed orange or grapefruit juice. It saves time and is quite palatable, although fresh is always preferable.

Sour milk and homemade kefir can also be considered natural chelators. They fight putrefaction by increasing the good intestinal flora and have been used in Bulgaria and other Balkan countries since ancient times. The large number of good bacteria in soured milk removes toxic matter from both the small and large intestine. The Russian biologist and scientist Elie Metchnikoff (1845-1916) researched different ways to prolong life. He came to the conclusion that it could happen by restricting the intake of meat to repress the growth of harmful bacteria and sowing our intestinal tract with lactic acid bacilli instead. Adding friendly microorganisms to our diet is a way to avoid a large number of diseases.

A musician friend of mine proved this theory. She had suffered from cancer years back. Although she managed to be in remission, the disease came back when she was in her eighties. At some point, she was so sick that she was unable to eat or drink anything but sour milk. She asked her friends to not spend their money on flowers but rather bring her yogurt and buttermilk instead. She lived exclusively on the sour milk for six weeks and then was back to normal. After the incident, she still lived for many years and entertained her friends with lovely piano concerts.

Eating nothing but yogurt and ground flax seeds alternating with black cherry juice might give you two, three, or even more abundant bowel movements a day. It will probably remain a mystery where all this "waste" comes from, but after a few days your skin will be glowing. You will lose weight and feel good all over.

Low fat cottage cheese instead of yogurt was used with great success by the world famous German physician, chemist, and physicist Dr. Johanna Budwig (1908-2003) for all kinds of ailments. She came up with a simple recipe that healed hundreds of people even in the last stages of cancer. The mixture helps with digestion and noticeably improves the appearance of skin and hair. In one of her books she also recommends her famous "cream" for people who suffer from arthritis, heart disease and other ailments. Her recipe seems almost too simple to have an effect on life threatening diseases but Dr. Budwig healed many people who were beyond hope. Although the Budwig cream was the main ingredient of her treatments, she also recommended a vegetarian diet and made a few other suggestions.

To prepare the cream, mix with an immersion blender six tablespoons of low fat cottage cheese with half the amount (three tablespoons) of flaxseed oil and a little bit of low fat milk until the ingredients acquire a creamy consistency. Then add two tablespoons of freshly ground flax seeds. It is optional to add Chia seeds, honey, fruit, and nuts later on. According to her research, Dr. Budwig claimed that the combination of oil and protein in its emulsified state creates a new substance, which heals and rejuvenates the body and is neither oil or protein.

Garlic is not everybody's favorite, but it is one of the most effective supplements in existence. Most people avoid it because of its unpleasant smell. Freshly squeezed lemon juice eliminates the problem. Garlic has been used since ancient times for all kinds of ailments. It is considered a natural antibiotic, believed to expel intestinal worms, lower bad cholesterol, and can be used as a remedy for heart problems. Garlic strengthens the immune system and is one of the best remedies for a cold or flu. Research has shown that it destroys cancer cells and is effective in its prevention. Garlic was used by the Romans, Egyptians, Greeks, and Israelites as a talisman to ward off evil. (Careful, it might ward off your significant other as well!) During the Middle Ages, people who ate garlic are reported to have survived the bubonic plague. Eaten in large quantities, garlic might be useful in the fight against AIDS due to its antiviral, antiseptic, and antibiotic properties. Garlic is another natural chelator, which cleans our blood vessels and improves circulation.

Years ago, a friend of mine asked me if I could recommend anything for her varicose veins. The lady was poor and often had nothing to eat at all. How could I suggest a diet for her? I lightly said, "Try eating garlic!" Months later, we met again and she thanked me profoundly for the wonderful remedy I had given her. I was confused. I had not given her anything. "Remember the varicose veins?" she said. "They were all over, and now they are gone." How many cloves did you eat?" I asked her. "Oh, about eighteen or twenty a day," she said. "Since you did not tell me how many, I ate as many as I could." She looked prettier than ever and there was no detectable smell. I have no idea for how long she ate garlic or how often. I only know that it seemed a miracle to see her like this. It must have pulled a lot of harmful substances out of her body.

There is no need to take this much garlic unless something really serious is going on and you want to get rid of it fast. One clove a day, chopped up for better absorption, should be enough to keep your immune system strong. It can be taken in the morning with a glass of water and lemon juice or in the evening before you go to bed.

Microwaved food seems to contribute to the formation of heavy metals in the body. It should be avoided at all costs. When you go to a restaurant and the plate with the food comes out hot, most likely it has been in the microwave oven. Better choose a different place next time, even if you have to wait a little longer for the food to be ready.

Eating at least once a day any of these chelators helps to clean our blood and keeps our immune system strong. It is worth it because healthy is beautiful. Whatever enters the body first, is more effective. Therefore, these special additions should be included in the first meal of the day. It gives protection. It is like going on a trip by car. Before we leave, we make sure there is gas in the tank and air in the tires. When we prepare ourselves, it is unlikely for emergencies to show up. In the same way our body responds with wellness when we give it the right food and water.

There is no need for us to understand all the details. Not even a doctor knows exactly what is going on inside of us but the body knows what to do. It cleanses and repairs itself continuously and lets us know when we don't support it. Our vital processes will be affected and disease shows up. Just as we create a disease, we can also learn to create health. We may have to try a few things and see how they work. Once we achieve results, nobody can convince us otherwise, because experience is the best teacher.

Mono Diets

Mono diets are a form of fasting or semi fasting. Due to their contents of fiber, organic water, vitamins and some minerals they are enormously cleansing. At the beginning of my own odyssey, I recovered very quickly from almost all of my health challenges by following mono diets. It meant eating only one kind of fruit alternating with chamomile tea. It changed my life. For cleansing, fruit is ideal but any kind of mono diet is beneficial, whether it be with juices, vegetables, rice or water only.

Here are a few of the benefits attributed to different fruits:

Apples	-	They strengthen our nervous system, normalize digestion, and improve liver function.
Papaya	-	is laxative, soothing for the stomach and intestine.
Pineapple	-	improves digestion and removes parasites. It dissolves fat cells, reduces swelling, fights inflammation and is disinfecting. Just like papaya, pineapple has a lot of enzymes.
Figs	-	are laxative and help to eliminate parasites.
Mangoes	-	are laxative, strengthen sexual glands and increase fertility.

Watermelon	-	is diuretic.
Cherries	-	are laxative, improve liver functioning, and lessen arthritis pain.
		Cherries are rich in organic iron.
Grapes	-	are diuretic, laxative, help in cases of rheumatism, arthritis, and gout. They are also believed to have anti-cancer properties, specially the dark kind.
Stewed Prunes	-	dissolve mucus and are very laxative.
Apricots	-	are some of the most rejuvenating fruits. They have lots of vitamin A and C and contain magnesium.
Oranges	-	are cleansing for the liver, laxative, and have a very alkalizing effect.
Limes/ Lemons	-	are blood cleansing, strengthen the liver, eliminate mucus, and improve nearly all physical functions. They are among the most healing fruits of all. (Always drink lemon juice with a straw to protect the enamel of your teeth.)

A young woman from a town in the Northern part of Mexico at the age of 23 was diagnosed with cancer in her uterus. She was told by the doctors that the cancer had spread and it was too late to operate. She started to read books on natural healing, followed diets with different kinds of fruit, took steam baths, did body wraps with clay, and eventually learned about the grape diet, which was thought to be particularly effective in cases of cancer. Not having much to lose, she started the diet the best she could, eating every day lots of grapes. After a year, she was cancer free, became pregnant, and later gave birth to a baby girl in the same hospital where two years earlier they had sent her home to die.

The pretty nurse from Costa Rica, mentioned earlier, also claims that she had been healed from cancer of the uterus by eating nothing but grapes and green leafy vegetables for six weeks.

One of my clients decided to eat papaya for two weeks. At the end of this time, she eliminated a huge worm. Apparently, the worm was not happy anymore inside of her due to the lack of other food.

Eating only rice, certain vegetables, or greens can be considered a mono diet as well, as long as you limit yourself to one particular kind of food. One of the most powerful mono diets seems to be that of the green leaf. A pretty young lady shared that after trying many different diets she now had found the most effective one of all: the green diet. She said that she had lost close to twenty pounds in a short time by eating only greens, and that she felt wonderful. She was eating salads and drinking nothing but green juices and smoothies. On the day I saw her she even wore a green dress to match her program.

It may not be necessary to eat this simple for longer periods of time to get results. When I started, I lived on one kind of fruit every fourth day and in less than two months I changed from a very sick person to one of vibrant health. Even one day a week with fruit can improve our state of health tremendously.

The key is always simplicity. We can go at our own pace, which means if even one whole day is too much for you, substituting one meal a day for fresh fruit or a salad may be a great alternative.

Oats for Beauty

Oats are among the healthiest gluten free grains on earth with many benefits. No wonder, they were the preferred cereal of the prophet Muhammad. You can eat them cooked as porridge or use them in a shake or muesli to benefit hair, skin and fingernails, to lose weight or get more energy. They also calm the nervous system, and you can use them in the evening to help you sleep better. Oats contain nearly all the B-vitamins as well as some vitamin E. They contain carbohydrates, fiber, fat and seven out of nine of the essential amino acids, which means their nutritional value is close to that of animal protein but without the toxins found in meat. Oats are filling and include the most important minerals: iron, magnesium, calcium, potassium, sodium, phosphorus, zinc, copper, manganese, and silica. In other words, oats contain so many nutrients you might want to eat them as a complete meal. They can be combined with dry fruit, nuts, seeds or even vegetables. You can cook them with bone broth, if you prefer, or add a little honey and cinnamon, or a pinch of unrefined sea salt. Soon you will notice their enormous rejuvenating effect. They can also be added to smoothies.

One way to ingest oats is to soak them overnight, maybe around three tablespoons, and in the morning blend them with apple or papaya, two tablespoons of ground flaxseeds and one tablespoon of Chia seeds. Honey can be added to taste, if desired. Of course, the flaxseeds and Chia seeds can also be added to cooked oatmeal or porridge. For those of us who find fasting with fruit or water difficult, we may try oats or porridge as a mono diet instead. They keep us full.

Oats improve digestion, give us energy during the day and help us sleep better at night. They help to regulate our weight. Those who are overweight will lose a few pounds and those who are too skinny will gain some. Eating oats regularly helps lower cholesterol, normalizes blood sugar, and some people say it even improves their sex life. British born Claude Stanley Choules (1901-2011) was one of the oldest men in Australia. He died at the age of 110, and his secret to a long life was to avoid all kinds of medication, eat a bowl of oatmeal every morning, drink fresh juices, and swim in the ocean, which he did till he was 100 years old. Although he served in the Navy, he became a pacifist and published his first book past the age of 100. He believed that oats and cod liver oil helped him stay youthful.

Dr. Miguel Pros, a physician in Spain, near Barcelona, has healed thousands of patients from all kind of diseases with a vegetarian regimen based on oats as their main ingredient to which fruit, and raw or cooked vegetables could be added. Not being much of a chef myself, I like the idea of eating oats because they are easy to prepare, still leaving the option to eat other things, if desired. Oats probably do more for health and youthfulness than expensive supplements. After searching for years for the ideal food, whether it is a fruit, greens, rice, or fish, I am now convinced that it may be oatmeal. They made me feel great when I "fasted" on oats for three days.

Oats are also used in beauty preparations or in bath water for softer skin and to get rid of eczema. The more you use them, the more benefits you will experience. If there is only one thing you want to take away from reading this book, it may be to include more oats in your diet.

Finding a Middle Way

If you have a significant other going into a different direction health-wise, like myself, you will understand that sometimes it is not easy to convince them of anything that might be good for them. I gave up making suggestions and instead decided to take better care of myself and teach by example. In fact, a miracle happened already. The significant other came up with some brilliant ideas, claiming them as his own. Perfect! I am proud of the changes he made and realize that it is difficult for somebody who is neither willing nor ready to give up anything. My loved one likes to eat, drink, dance and be merry. He is far from going on a diet, and a colonic irrigation is something he definitely will not consider. I do understand that part. He also believes that fasting, cleansing and raw food are for crazy people only.

Of course, he cannot be counted among the healthy ones but hours of daily walking and dancing make up for his poor diet. As long as he has no pain and there are medical doctors to take care of him, he is happy and we hope for the best.

What we eat on a daily basis makes a lot of difference, especially in the long run. When you love somebody, you want the best for them. You want to be with them without having to worry whether they make it through their next surgery. Of course, the significant other would love to be healthy. The problem is that he has the illusion that he can continue eating what he has always eaten, expecting a miracle to happen or that the doctor can fix it.

It is important to find common ground with our partner. Sometimes we have to make concessions. Don't be too hard on either one of you and always take care of yourself first. Nobody is perfect and we all do what we think is best. Then gradually include more fresh juices and vegetables in the menu. Both of you benefit when you reduce the amount of meat and desserts. When we do something with love, it will be felt. The other person will either appreciate it or at least go along with the program, especially if after awhile it makes them feel better. It is not about being vegan, fruitarian, or a meat eater. It is about being healthy and enjoying life together.

A person who does not overeat and includes some kind of exercise in their activities will experience no harm with fish, eggs or poultry in their diet. Wine and beer are less harmful than soft drinks, particularly the "diet" kind with artificial sweeteners, and in moderate amounts alcohol can even be beneficial. There is no need to convince somebody of a heroic plan, much less to ask your partner to eat something they do not like. Going at his own pace, he may reach his goals faster than expected.

According to a research published in *National Geographic* on areas where people live the longest and are active to an advanced age, the majority are not vegetarian, although the fittest ones eat very little meat. Studies on a large scale are more enlightening. For instance, the Adventists are well known for their good health and longevity. Many of them are still physically active between ninety and 100 years of age. Those who are vegetarians tend to have less cholesterol, less diabetes, and in general a more normal blood pressure than their meat-eating peers. One study also shows that vegans on the average weigh thirty pounds less than meat eaters.

Another study carried out by Loma Linda University in 2012 included 96,000 men and women of all ethnicities from the

U.S. and Canada. They were divided into four groups: meat eaters, ovo-lacto vegetarians (people who consume eggs and dairy), vegans, and pesco-vegetarians, i.e. people who eat a plant-based diet with up to one serving of fish per day. The meat eaters weighed on the average twenty pounds more than people from the other groups and were likely to die sooner. The people in the fourth group seemed to live the longest, which seems to indicate that this diet, rich in organic vegetables, with some fruit, fish, and oils in moderation, may give the best results, especially when combined with exercise. It is a diet that not only keeps us healthy but also helps us to stay close to our ideal weight.

People in other Blue Zones have similar diets: most of them eat about 90 percent plant-based food and the rest is divided between fruit, fish, eggs, cheese, or chicken. Healthy oils in small amounts are included as well. The main ingredients in a diet recommended by Adventists are avocados, salmon, nuts, beans, water, oatmeal, whole grain sourdough bread, and soymilk.

Whether a diet is raw or cooked, vegetarian, or includes animal protein, the most important point is to keep it simple. As long as we do not overeat or mix too many ingredients in one meal, we are all right. Dr. Hiromi Shinya, a famous Japanese-American surgeon and gastroenterologist in New York, has helped thousands of patients return to health through diet. He wrote two life-changing books and recommends a diet with 85 percent plant-based food and only fifteen percent animal food. In his opinion, brown rice and small fish are the best foods. He recommends using unrefined salt, some fruit, an enzyme rich juice made with green, leafy vegetables, as well as occasional fasting. Since our soils are mineral depleted, he is much in favor of taking extra supplements and he is not against occasional colonics or enemas in order to achieve maximum health.

Dr. Shinya's recommendations can be followed by almost anyone without the need to go to extremes or live on raw food only. He suggests though that we get our enzymes from fresh fruit and vegetables. Simplicity is important. Eating a variety of food like soup, salad, potatoes, meat, dessert, coffee, wine and beer all at the same time, has negative effects and the body will respond with disease. With aches and pains, nausea, digestive issues, and weight gain, the body clearly alerts us that something needs to be changed, unless we want to get worse.

Then there are "silent" diseases, like cancer, with no pain, where previous symptoms might have been suppressed repeatedly. In heart disease, the reaction can be sudden. We need to pay more attention to small warning signs when almost all symptoms can still be reversed. Unfortunately, most people believe they can eat just about anything without consequences, and whatever shows up later is pure coincidence.

A study published in the *Lancet Medical Journal* shows that 20 percent of early deaths are diet related. Toxic food ingredients, added sugar, pesticides, artificial color or flavor, antibiotics, preservatives and heavy metals, are not ignored by the body. We may be able to tolerate them for a while, but in the long run they lead to disease, premature aging and in some cases even death. When we go and see a physician for our problems, he or she prescribes medication, and in some cases suggests surgery. Although necessary in an emergency, all medication and procedures have side effects. They disturb the natural harmony in our body. Healing comes from the inside. Our main goal must be to restore harmony, which is mainly done through a healthy lifestyle, diet being an important part of it.

What Is Holding You Back?

In the Orient there is a belief that we are rich in proportion to what we can do without. This applies to many areas of our life, not only to our physical or financial state of affairs. By giving up certain foods, our health will improve but there are other areas that want improvement as well. If there is anything that we know is harmful to us and we still can't give it up, we are addicted to it. It is holding us back from reaching our full potential.

By now we already know that our food should be of the highest quality, meaning that it should be as unprocessed as possible and full of nutrients. In such case even small amounts of food might be sufficient. Actually, small amounts are preferable. Dr. Amen Ra, by many considered the strongest man in the world, eats only one vegan meal a day and proves the point.

None of the great saints and sages are known for their opulent meals. They either temporarily abstained from food altogether or ate very little. In fact, the sicker people are, the hungrier they seem to be. Often, they make trips to the refrigerator in the middle of the night, because they feel they still need more food. It is not the amount of food we eat that counts but rather what part of it is being absorbed. Our body does need vitamins, minerals, fat and protein to function properly, just like a car needs gasoline. However, when we have become a host to harmful microorganisms and we start feeling weak and tired, we crave coffee, sugar or other stimulants to bring our energy back. The result may be just the opposite. Instead of getting our strength back, our body will gradually deteriorate and show signs of aging way ahead of time. We may become addicted, thereby initiating a never-ending cycle. If coffee and candies are not enough, we may reach for cigarettes and alcohol. None of them are a long-term solution to our problems.

Sometimes we are not even aware of the fact that we have become addicted. It does not always have to be alcohol or an illegal drug. We might be addicted to our morning coffee, to chocolates, to diet food, soft drinks, to overmedicating ourselves, to work, to sleeping too much, to clutter, sex, or a toxic relationship. If we cannot live without them, knowing that they do nothing to improve the quality of our lives, then we have become addicted. These addictions are holding us back from leading the life we would like to have.

The first step to do something about it, may be to realize that we need to change something. Even keeping clutter in our surroundings may be a form of addiction. Things we have not used for a year or two, collect dust. Anything we do not use, that is dirty, needs repair, or belongs to somebody else, makes the energy stagnant and prevents us from progressing. We might not see the relationship between having everything in order and moving on to something better, but it is definitely there. Clutter may affect our health, our finances, and our relationships. One way to move on could be to look at the details, getting rid of everything that does not serve us anymore. There may be clutter in our home, in our car, or our finances. Then start to make improvements. Problems related to our health may be related to the food we eat and toxic matter inside of us. Fasting and cleansing may be the answer to get our circulation going again. Make better choices in the future.

In your home, get rid of anything you do not need anymore. Giving things away is only half of the equation. The other part is cleaning and blessing whatever stays. We can make our home more beautiful with flowers, pictures, a few new cushions, or whatever comes to mind. It does not have to cost much. To do the whole house in one session is overwhelming. Start with one small area, like a drawer. Then go into another room that needs improvement. It could be the kitchen cabinets, the refrigerator, then the bathroom, the bedroom, and eventually the garage. Wouldn't it lift your spirits if you replaced the old sheets for fresh ones? Don't forget to look through your handbag or to balance your checkbook. The car needs to be clean and in good condition. Does it need service? When you are done, everything should look neat and inviting. It should give you pleasure to live in such nice surroundings.

Whatever is not needed, give it away. You will not need it again and bless whatever is left. It will make a huge difference in your life. It allows greater good to come to you.

Whenever I am not sure what to do next, I start to clean. Clothes go to Goodwill, old cosmetics go in the trash. The same with vitamin bottles, shoes I have not worn for some time, things I bought on sale and can't even remember why I have them. Years ago, when I moved into my new home, it was a great opportunity to only take with me what I really wanted. I packed everything into boxes, and before I decided whether to keep something or get rid of it, my motto was: "In case of doubt, throw it out!" I have never regretted doing it.

A few days ago, I threw away an old soap dish and gave some suits that belonged to my deceased husband to Goodwill. I also cleaned out a drawer. It is amazing how such simple changes made me feel freer, and my energy has increased too. I am now ready for more adventures. Coincidence? I am looking forward to giving away more stuff and see what other blessings will come to me.

Sometimes we are so attached to certain items that we don't even realize we have outgrown them a long time ago. It may be certain kinds of food, old souvenirs, or toxic relationships.

There is no purpose in holding on to them. It is best to let go of whatever is negative and brings our energy down. As long as we hang on to what does not serve us, nothing better can come in.

Our physical body is very much part of the cleaning process. In order to allow for better health, we need to get rid of toxins. Vitamins and minerals cannot work well in a toxic body. It is a good sign when more stuff goes out than we take in. As soon as we eat less or fast for a day or longer, the weaker, older and sick cells are eliminated and then are gradually replaced by new ones. Over 70 percent of our stools are bacteria and dead cells, something we don't want in our body. After doing a cleanse, food will be absorbed much better and we only need smaller amounts. Also, the body becomes aware of harmful substances faster and lets us know about them. It is all about the quality and not quantity in our lives.

Sometimes we keep items we do not need or acquire even more stuff. We believe that the next piece of jewelry, more money in the bank, working extra hours, or finding another partner will bring us the happiness we have been looking for. People say that happiness is like a butterfly. When we chase it, it flies away, and when we stay still, it might come and rest on our shoulder. So, take more time to enjoy life. The rest takes care on its own.

Sugar might be our greatest enemy. Over consumption can have dire consequences. It may give us a temporary high, but it does not bring us happiness in the long run. Recent studies revealed that it ages the brain and there might be a link between sugar consumption and Alzheimer's disease.

To give up sugar can be a challenge. It is believed to be more addictive than cocaine. Repetitive fasting and a lot of will power may help overcome the temptation. Increasing temporarily the amount of fats and protein in our diet may help as well. Food in general can be an addiction. Studies have shown that the greater the gap between meals, the less the body will be depleted. Fasting is the one thing that most replenishes our life force. It is a form of inner cleaning, which regenerates our energy. We will live longer and be healthier. Intermittent fasting or instead, living one day a week on fruit, water or one kind of food only, can be most beneficial. The less we eat and the simpler our meals, the more energy will be available for healing, and ultimately, for the creation of beauty.

Other addictions may be caffeine and overeating in general. All of them create a high degree of acidity, which makes the absorption of oxygen and minerals more difficult.

Poor people, who eat less, seem to be healthier than those who can afford luxuries. An acquaintance of mine, a young man in Mexico City, told me how he and his entire family lived for two years on nothing but corn tortillas and chilies. No milk, no meat, no candies, no soft drinks, nothing else! The young man was the image of health and beauty, tall, with an athletic countenance, beautiful thick black, curly hair, white teeth and a smooth complexion. He told me that he grew up in a village in the North of the country. At one time, there was a drought and he, his mother, and five siblings, had nothing to eat. They survived on this meager diet of corn tortillas and chilies for two years. Did they look malnourished? On the contrary! I hardly ever saw more beautiful people than this family.

Eating meat is not an addiction, but in large amounts it is harmful to the body. It may even cause colon cancer. Some people prefer to eat very little meat or none at all, to spare the animals. Animals have feelings. Our pets are unconditional love. Cows, horses, elephants and chimpanzees stay close to their offspring, and ducks and swans on a lake travel together as a family. You can see there is a bond between them. Some animals are in mourning when their companion dies and refuse to eat. Many spiritually oriented people and great teachers like Socrates, Pythagoras, Ovid, Tolstoy, Tesla and others opted for a vegetarian lifestyle.

There is no need to give up everything we enjoy. The problem arises when our food, medication, or "friends" become harmful to us. We are addicted when in spite of being aware of it, we keep them around. Whether it is an illegal drug or living without cigarettes, coffee, candy or donuts, if being without them makes you miserable, you are addicted. They keep you from living your whole potential. The easiest way to determine what you want in your life in the future, what makes you feel better, is to start with your surroundings, i.e. clearing clutter. Then you follow with a plan for your health. The more you eliminate, the better you will feel. After awhile it gets easier. You get a feeling of accomplishment. You start feeling better and you know you want to go even further. You see more clearly what is best for you. Every time you clean something out, your wellbeing increases. You become the best you can be, and more blessings will come into your life. You get closer to living your full potential and eventually you see that YOU are the most important person in your life.

New Habits for a Better Life

Any change we make has to be repeated over a certain period of time in order to produce results. In other words, we have to create new habits. Doing something once will not have much effect, unless you take cyanide. In that case, one dose might be enough. Eating healthy for a day or two makes no difference in our degree of well-being. If we generally follow a good diet, our immune system will be strong and even a little spoiled food or medication will only show temporary adverse effects.

We looked at people who turned their life around. They did something differently than what they used to do before. They either replaced an old habit or added something new to their current lifestyle. In either case, it is important to be persistent with something that works. People often pray to God for something. They ask for a better job, a new partner, a pay raise, peace of mind, getting out of debt, or improved health. Whatever it may be, if we keep doing the same things, there won't be much change. We keep going in the same direction, regardless of how much we pray. There is a saying: "Only a fool keeps doing the same things and expects different results."

Changing our lifestyle altogether may be scary because we don't know what to expect. Taking one step at a time is another option. If it works, we continue, and if it doesn't we let it go.

Following are a few examples of people who implemented one or two minor changes at a time with great success and then decided to stay with them.

There is Janet, who managed to transform herself from being sick and stressed into a happy and healthy person. Looking at her now, you would say she is one of the healthiest women you have ever met. Years back, she suffered from cancer in her uterus and underwent a complete hysterectomy. She used to be the CEO of a big corporation. Her second unhappy marriage also ended in divorce. She had a very stressful life. There was tension at home and at the office. In her position, she was required to dress formally, wear make-up on a daily basis, and show a happy attitude towards customers, regardless of what she was going through or how she felt inside. For Janet, her cancer turned out to be a blessing. She had come to a point where she could not stand the pressure any more. Although materially she was well off, the life she was leading was far from ideal. She lived in a nice house, drove a big car and judging from the outside, she had everything she could wish for.

Right after her surgery she was unable to go back to the office and had to rest. Being used to an active life, staying at home was not fulfilling. She started reading books on health and metaphysics, and in order to make some money she gave readings and shared her knowledge of metaphysics. The more she did it, the more she liked it. Most of all, she now had an opportunity to lead a stress-free life. She decided to resign from her position at the company and to redo her life. The first thing she did was improve her diet. She included a lot of salads and more raw food. She also bought a Colema Board for home colonics.

Then Janet started jogging and followed her newly found hobbies of reading and metaphysics. She then decided to take a job at a wholesale produce company, where she could dress informally and did not experience the pressure she had before. Gradually, her health turned around and the cancer stayed behind. With dedication, exercise, self-discipline, and a spiritually oriented life she became one of the healthiest persons you can imagine. Eventually, she met her third husband and moved with him to Hawaii, where they are, hopefully, still living happily together.

The story sounds like a fairy tale, and in a way it is. Once Janet acquired new habits, she managed to turn her life around and recovered from a very serious illness. It also shows that the changes can be simple. The sooner we start, the more successful we will be. Although diet is important, improvements in other areas count as well. For instance, a daily walk in the open air dissipates negative energy or inspires us to follow other activities. Reading, writing, music, painting, practicing some sport or spending time with a pet or a loved one can bring us joy and give our life a new direction.

There is not one formula that works for everybody. We have to consider our age, environment, climate, occupation, preferences, and financial situation. As a general rule for physical wellbeing Hippocrates' recommendation from 2,500 years ago is still valid. He said: "May thy food be thy medicine and thy medicine thy only food." Whatever we put in our body forms our blood, our tissues, and organs. There is no reason to not feel good.

Without falling prey to major illness, a few other friends have created a healthy and successful life for themselves. All they invested was their willingness to take their next step.

Gloria is one of them. She works in a government office. In spite of a busy day she has her life together. She is vegetarian, practices half an hour of yoga every day and, courageous as she is, uses only cold water for her showers all year round. Cold showers activate our circulation and Gloria never feels tired. Getting into the shower is quite a challenge. To be honest, I only tried it for a few days because I promised that I would do it. Although I felt wonderful afterwards, I prefer to use warm water first and then rinse with cold water afterwards.

Mrs. Leroy is another one of my heroes. As the mother of a famous actor and head of a huge household, she has many social commitments. She still likes to keep her life simple and supports a number of charitable causes. Years back, she joined my yoga classes and I was surprised how young she looked. Being around thirty myself at the time, I would have guessed her age to be around thirty-five or maximum forty. Her body was slender and strong. She had neither wrinkles nor gray hair. I was more than surprised when she told me that she was sixty-five.

On one occasion, she invited me to her home and we spent time in her beautiful garden. She offered me a glass of juice, and then reached for a telephone in one of the trees to ask for it from the kitchen. A telephone in the garden to talk to the kitchen! Well, I was impressed again. We talked about lifestyles and apart from frugal eating habits and a love for outdoor activities like tennis and gardening, I could not pinpoint what Mrs. Leroy's secret might be. Later she told me that as a devout Catholic during Lent she lived exclusively on oatmeal for forty days, something she had done as long as she could remember. Her practice reminded me of Dr. Sperl, who even in his nineties had the blood of a young man. He too lived an entire month on nothing but mangos every spring.

My neighbor Aby just reached sixty. Everybody envies her slender body and inexhaustible energy. With two jobs, she is also one of the busiest people I know. She gets up early in the morning to take care of her husband, who leaves for work around 6:00 a.m. She then walks her dog for half an hour, and twice a week spends another thirty minutes at the gym before she starts her work day. She is always cheerful. If you ever need a friend, she will be there for you. Her secret? She eats lots of salads with a little protein at dinner time, and she has the willpower to stay away from sweets.

Another person who added a few changes to his daily routine is a fifty-six-year-old truck driver. He used to struggle with being overweight. Since he mostly eats at truck stops and has to get his freight to its destination as fast as possible, he does not give himself the time to walk or enjoy healthy meals. Without being aware of it, he suffered from Candida, which was one of the reasons he could not lose weight. Once we addressed the problem, Mr. A. dropped about fifty pounds in three months and kept the weight off. Due to his work, it was not easy for him to change his eating habits, but he went from 100 percent junk food to some salads and protein. In addition, he buys ground flax seeds at a health food store and mixes two tablespoons of them with water or juice, which he then drinks morning and evening. This beverage keeps him regular giving him several bowel movements a day. The second thing he does is eat four cloves of chopped garlic every day, followed by the juice of several limes or lemons. The lemon juice eliminates the smell and in spite of this massive dosage of garlic he manages to keep his friends. There is no way this man can get sick!

One of my clients in her sixties started out with different health challenges. In the beginning, her face had a yellowish tint and her eyes showed a lot of red blood vessels. She ate fruit before each meal and drank green smoothies in the morning, made from spinach, parsley, cucumber, sprouts, and some fruit. Two years later she looked like in her forties. All wrinkles had disappeared and the yellowish skin tone had changed to rosy.

Perfection probably remains an illusion. How close we get to it, is beyond our control. All we can do for our health is follow the best possible diet and do it consistently.

Rabindranath Tagore, one of India's most outstanding poets, describes our plight perfectly. His story is about a man who has been looking for God all his life. One day he comes to a house with a sign on the door which says: "Here lives God." He was surprised and wondered if this could be true. If he found God, then all his journeys, his adventures, the longing, his theories, promises, pilgrimages, they all would come to an end. He started running. The story goes that he still keeps searching but he avoids that particular house so he can keep seeking.

It is our journeys that make life interesting. It is our seeking, searching, making mistakes, then moving on in spite of obstacles; all the time trying to find different ways to reach happiness. There is always hope to attain what we are looking for. It is called life. Our desire gives us opportunities to explore new avenues. Whether we are looking for more money, possessions, better health, love, joy, or peace, we do our best to obtain them. Sometimes the goal seems to be really close but we never seem to reach it. There is always more. Happiness is elusive, so we sacrifice a little more. We grow and try to become a better person. We explore other options. Maybe the key is in working harder and having more, or it is in having less. Maybe we should sacrifice something. Maybe it is in helping others. Maybe we need to improve our eating habits or start tithing. Let your imagination fly. There is not one way that is for everybody but whatever we do, it will bring us a step closer to where we want to be.

Sometimes we have to do things nobody else has done before. A hundred years ago, flying across the ocean seemed impossible. Yet, Charles Lindbergh thought of it. On May 12, 1927, he was the first person to cross the Atlantic Ocean in a non-stop flight. Without Thomas Alba Edison we would not have the light bulb. Although it is said that he failed nine hundred ninety-nine times, he never thought of them as failures. He kept trying and was sure that each "failure" brought him closer to success. Once we find something that works, others may even decide to follow in our footsteps.

One of these persons was Mr. Allan Taylor from England, who cured himself of cancer at the age of seventy-eight. After a surgery, which removed nine inches of his colon, followed by three months of chemotherapy, Mr. Taylor received a letter from the hospital in April 2012, stating that neither chemotherapy nor any other surgery would be of help to him and that nothing else could be done to prevent his death. Mr. Taylor did not take their word for it. Since no more help could be expected in the traditional way, he searched for alternative therapies on the internet. After four months on a new diet and another check-up in the same hospital, on August 6, 2012, he received confirmation that there was no trace of cancer in his body anymore.

Mr. Taylor followed some simple steps: He avoided red meat and all dairy products. Instead, he consumed plenty of fresh fruit and vegetables every day. He also mixed a teaspoon of barley grass powder into a glass of hot water twice a day, which he believed greatly contributed to his recovery. He also added a few other supplements to his diet like apricot kernels, kelp, and vitamin C and included more raw food. He thereby created a high pH in his body, knowing that cancer cells cannot survive in an alkaline environment. He did what he thought was best and says that now he feels like twenty-one again. At the time he took his health in his own hands all medical treatments were discontinued.

By following Nature's ways, we follow God's ways, and God's ways are simple. What these people did was change their diet, exercise and use a few key supplements.

Questions and Answers

Whenever we start something new, there is uncertainty. It is a challenge. Even if a program or a diet may have worked for thousands of people, there are no two people exactly alike. I used to wonder whether certain changes would be helpful to me, because my problem was different from those of others. And yet, we also have a lot in common.

Naturopathy does not address any particular disease. In fact, the name of a disease does not matter at all. It is only a label for a combination of symptoms. Natural healing or naturopathy is about cleansing and strengthening all organs. It is a kind of purification.

After detoxification, our energy usually returns and unwanted symptoms disappear. It is as if we grow younger, stronger, and healthier. Somebody with multiple challenges will often see them go away completely. Doubts tend to appear at the time of a healing crisis when the body brings unwanted stuff to the surface. It might be in the form of a cold, a fever, skin rashes, phlegm, diarrhea, restlessness, feeling tired or irritable. The bad stuff is trying to leave the body, just like in a house cleaning. Those are the times when many lose faith and go back to their physicians. Medication will stuff the toxins back into the system. We might initially feel better because elimination has stopped, but the body will make other efforts to purify itself before it can return to health.

I am not a medical doctor, and all I can do is share my own views and experience regarding some of the most frequently asked questions. These ideas might be quite different from what you have heard before:

1. Heredity

People often are fearful that they might get a disease, especially cancer or diabetes, because either their parents or grandparents had it. My answer is that we do not inherit a disease. We inherit our height, the color of our skin, hair, eyes, and maybe our bone structure. As far as disease is concerned, all we inherit is a tendency towards it.

Let's take diabetes as an example. It is a disease of the pancreas. If both our parents had it, most likely we will inherit a weakness of this particular organ. If only one parent suffered from diabetes and the other parent does not, then the children may or may not get the disease. To make it easier to understand, let's take hair color. If the mother was blonde and the father dark haired, then any of the siblings will be born either blonde, dark haired, or with a color in between. In the same way, if one parent has diabetes and the other one does not, the children **may** inherit an insufficiency of the pancreas. However, since the body renews itself, there is a good possibility that the organ in question completely regenerates and the disease never shows up or heals itself at a later date, provided we choose a better lifestyle.

2. Why am I always hungry?

This happens to many of us. We are hungry and then reach for "comfort food" instead of a real meal. Comfort foods are little snacks with hardly any nutritional value. Temporarily they give us a little more energy. We crave them due to a lack of real nutrients. Our body needs vitamins, minerals, protein, and healthy oils to function well. When parasites, fungus, mold, yeast and other toxins are present, they prevent proper absorption of nutrients, and when the body is deficient in vital substances, it lets us know. We feel tired or hungry, sometimes both. Sweets bring our energy up quickly but then it plummets even more afterwards, so we have to keep eating. Once we get rid of toxic matter, the body is able to absorb nutrients properly and the cravings and excessive appetite will stop.

3. What can I do about a cold?

A cold is one of the body's desperate ways to rid itself of toxins. It can be prevented through inner cleansing. Once we have a cold, we should not fight it, but rather support the body in its detoxification process with rest, lemon juice, garlic, or hot teas. Colds are falsely attributed to bad weather, but it is the body's way to eliminate toxins. When people get sick at the beginning of the year they blame it on the weather. They do not realize that most likely they have been overeating during the holidays. If we decide to take care of a cold naturally, we will feel much cleaner and clearer afterwards and probably not get another cold for a very long time. Strengthening the immune system is one of the best ways to prevent a cold.

Flu shots might prevent unpleasant symptoms, but they can create something worse later on. A cold with all its symptoms like pain, fever, and headaches that make us feel miserable, is a form of purification. The body tries to eliminate all kinds of toxins, including residues of medication. Since there is contamination everywhere, i.e. in the air we breathe, the water, our food, and things we come in contact with, a form of purification is actually needed occasionally. If we know how to take care of ourselves and remain moderate in our eating habits, the symptoms will be rather mild and easy to deal with. I usually take a hot bath, drink freshly squeezed orange juice with plenty of garlic chopped up, and the problem will be over within a day or two.

Getting sick is not about bugs; it is about the terrain. When our blood is clean and our body does not have a lot of toxins to eliminate, our immune system will be strong and we feel good. Professor Arnold Ehret proved this theory when he spent time among people with cholera after he crossed the Alps into Italy. He and his companion fasted before the enterprise and neither one of them contracted the disease. If the body is toxic and their immune system weak, people can die from a serious cold. Others don't get it at all, being exposed to the same environment.

4. Should I use salt?

Our blood is similar in its composition to ocean water, and ocean water is salty. Without salt, the water would putrefy. This does not necessarily mean that we have to consume salt. In fact, many medical doctors prescribe diets without salt, especially for patients with high blood pressure. Salt tends to increase water retention.

We need to be aware of the fact that there are two kinds of salt. In ancient times, salt was highly appreciated. It was considered more valuable than gold. Salaries were paid in salt. Today it is shunned. The salt referred to in Biblical times was unrefined and full of minerals, quite different from the white table salt we find today in our supermarkets, and which is nothing but sodium chloride with all other minerals taken out. Unrefined salt, like the pink Himalayan salt or grey Celtic salt, contains close to a hundred minerals, among them magnesium, which should not raise blood pressure in any way. Refined white salt is indeed detrimental to our health.

Out of fear, and due to health concerns, some people prefer the bland taste of food without salt. Monitor yourself for a few days and see whether raw, unrefined sea salt affects your blood pressure or whether the problem is due to something else. In one of the workshops I attended, a gentleman got up and shared that for many years he strictly avoided all salt and fat in order to keep his blood pressure in check and that he took medication for his condition. Finally, he disregarded these restrictions. To his surprise, his health and his blood pressure improved within a very short time, and he did not need his medication.

5. Which are the best healers?

A pleasant way to get well is to let others do some of the work for us. Massage therapists, acupuncturists, Reiki practitioners, nutritionists, colon therapists, and all holistic healers are excellent choices. Even psychics can be accurate in pinpointing the cause and location of a problem. Computers can give amazingly accurate information regarding physical, emotional or spiritual issues. However, we still have to do the main work ourselves with diet, fasting, and exercise. Problems let us know when we are off course and that we need to change something. They are there to teach us something and help us grow. By changing our diet, our blood values will change. Blood sugar, blood pressure, cholesterol, triglycerides, platelet count and whatever else reflects our state of health, most of the time will go back to optimal ranges afterwards.

6. How can I lose weight?

We relate a slim body to high energy and youthfulness. Therefore, in our culture almost everybody wants to lose weight. A weight problem is a health problem, often related to Candida overgrowth. By getting rid of Candida, the weight tends to come off by itself. An acquaintance of mine lost twenty-five pounds in three weeks simply by getting rid of the fungus. He had tried everything else before and nothing seemed to work. He started taking probiotics and a targeted supplement, avoided temporarily all kinds of sugar, caffeine, bread with yeast in it, alcohol, and fermented foods, and in less than a month he dropped the excess weight and his energy came back. He also slept better. All these symptoms were related to

Candida. Once the fungus is gone, one can eat fruit again, use healthy sweeteners like honey, Stevia or molasses, and bread in moderation, without gaining the weight back.

7. What can I do to sleep better?

Younger people have no problem sleeping. As we get older, for many it becomes more difficult to fall asleep or to sleep all night through. With advanced age, we actually need fewer hours of sleep, maybe around five or six hours are sufficient. So, don't worry if you don't sleep eight hours anymore.

I would try a bowl of oatmeal in the evening. Both its B-vitamins and minerals like calcium and magnesium strengthen the nervous system. A cup of chamomile tea or a warm tubby bath also help to promote restful sleep. Drinking a glass of wine occasionally helps to relax and may promote better sleep.

Something that works for me: I dissolve a teaspoon of apple cider vinegar with ¼ of a teaspoon of baking soda in half a glass of warm water and drink it before bedtime. Blackstrap molasses, honey, turmeric or cayenne pepper may be added, if desired.

8. Does fat make me fat?

There are bad fats and those which the body needs. Eating fat does not make us fat. In fact, healthy fats might even help us lose weight, since they give us a feeling of satiation. They stay longer in the body. Eskimos eat a lot of raw fat and maintain the weight appropriate for their body type. More and more researchers have come to the conclusion that not fat but sugar may be the culprit for excessive weight gain. Some healthy fats are extra virgin olive oil, hemp oil, flax seed oil, or coconut oil. They are health promoting, especially in their raw and unrefined state. Trans-fats on the other hand, like in heated animal fat, fried foods or margarine, can be quite harmful, especially for the heart. Fish oil and krill oil, taken as supplements, may help the body to lower cholesterol and improve skin health and eyesight. The best fats for cooking are coconut oil or ghee, both of which tolerate high temperatures without side effects.

9. How soon will I see results?

This is a question everybody wants an answer to. We wish it would happen overnight. Reversing symptoms is a process, and the time it takes to see results varies in each person. Age is one of the factors involved. Younger people heal faster. Medication can stay up to twenty years in our system and is difficult to eliminate. All chemicals and heavy metals are tenacious. Another factor is how far the illness has progressed and how willing are we to make changes. Our body forms new cells every day according to the food we eat, the air we breathe and the thoughts we think. Changes occur continuously, either for the better or for the worse. A return to health is often about cleansing. Once the majority of toxins are eliminated, the way we feel will be worth the effort. It is an investment in ourselves.

Since we are responsible for our own wellbeing, the question comes up whether we need medical doctors at all. Prevention is always the best medicine and before seeing any trained physician, my own choice would be to try Dr. Diet, Dr. Quiet, and Dr. Merryman first. However, if we waited too long or in an emergency we all need professional help.

Transformation

Several years ago, I heard a beautiful story. It is about an archer who eventually became king, probably in ancient India.

The king wanted to find a worthy successor for his throne, so he organized a contest and promised that the most skillful archer in the country would get half of his kingdom and the hand of this daughter in marriage. Among the participants was a man who was a thief, a liar, a cheater, and a murderer but it just so happened that he won the contest. With his victory, he was entitled to half the kingdom and to marry the princess. Instead of being full of joy, he got scared. What if somebody found out that he had been evil all his life? Instead of giving him the kingdom and betroth him to his daughter, in all likelihood the king would behead him. On the other hand, if he refused to marry, his chances to be hanged were just as good. What to do? The archer was in a serious plight.

He sent word to the princess and asked for her permission to postpone the wedding for two years. In the meantime, he went to the best mask maker he could find and asked him to fabricate a special mask for him, one that showed him smiling and happy. The mask maker was so skillful that the mask he produced was lifelike; nobody could tell the difference. The archer wore it day and night, fearful to take it off and that somebody would recognize him. With a happy smile on his face, it was impossible to behave mean and violent. He pretended to be kind and gentle, patient, caring, and generous. He won the hearts of the people and gradually the word got around that this man would be the king's son-in-law.

At the end of the two years he had to keep his promise and confront the princess. Whether he kept hiding or she found out, the future did not look too bright for him. When they met, he got all his courage together and said: "I have a confession to make. I am not the man you think I am. All this time I have been wearing a mask to hide my real Self, because I was afraid your father would behead me if he recognized me for who I am. You decide whether you want to go ahead with the wedding or not. He then took off his mask. For a few moments, the princess was speechless. All she could see was a beautiful human being, a man who was kind, loving, honest, patient, and generous, a man worthy of the kingdom. Finally, she said: "I don't know what you are talking about. You are far more beautiful than the mask you have been wearing."

During those two years the archer treated everybody with honesty and kindness and these traits became second nature to him. Indeed, he had become a new person.

Sometimes we too may find ourselves in a desperate situation. We made mistakes in the past and there are things we are not too proud of. It is impossible to change the past but we can do our best to create a better future. It takes courage and effort and the results may not appear overnight, but it can be done. We have to keep trying. As long as we hide our shortcomings, there cannot be true happiness. Every problem is a challenge we can overcome.

There are many ways to improve our health and our lives. One of them is through discipline. My Indian yoga master recommended that all disciples followed certain disciplines during the week between Christmas and the New Year, with the purpose to start January in perfect health. Besides, many believe that December is the month where the angels are closer to earth and our prayers are more effective. His suggestions are not easy to follow, because some of us work and others have social commitments. Of course, any other time of the year brings benefits as well.

Swami suggested we eat only one meal a day, preferably vegetarian. He also recommended one hour of yoga or other exercise, one hour for reading the Scriptures and another hour for meditation. Eating only one meal a day, and not necessarily vegetarian, is a good start. During the rest of the day one may eat fruit. Walking outdoors or practicing some other form of exercise, brings additional benefits. Reading the Scriptures, whether it is the Bible, the Koran, the Bhagavad Gita, the Course of Miracles, or any other teaching of the Masters, also attracts blessings. Prayer and meditation are also tools to progress on our spiritual path, even if only practiced for a few minutes every day. Prayer is asking God for favors and meditation is waiting for His answers. You may be surprised how peaceful you feel after a time in silence. Perhaps you find a solution to your problems or they disappear altogether.

In today's hectic lifestyle, prayer and meditation are more important than ever. As Leonard Cohen mentioned in one of his songs, "If we forget to pray to the Angels, the Angels forget to pray for us." If you want help from above, don't forget to pray.

Something else to consider for our well-being is our financial health. A lack of money can cause tremendous stress in other areas of our lives as well. It can affect our physical health, our relationships, our emotions, and everything else. One of the most effective ways to increase our wealth is to put aside 10 percent of our income. We can either give it to the source of our spiritual nourishment or create a Money Magnet. Every time you receive an increase, give 10 percent away to support something you want more of, or put it aside for yourself. The money in your magnet is not to be spent. The more it accumulates, the faster it will pull money towards you. It may come through your work, gifts, or other opportunities. The Money Magnet makes you rich. No matter how bad things may appear to be, when you know there is money in your magnet, you simply cannot feel poor. Your consciousness of wealth will make you act differently. You will probably be more generous, and you attract more good towards you. If 10 percent seems too much in the beginning, start with less. Ten is the magic number, and gradually you will build prosperity in all areas. Even your health and your relationships will improve.

The Blessings Are in the Journey

L ife itself is our greatest gift, and every day is a new beginning. Every day brings us new opportunities either to leave the past behind and create something different or, if things are going well, to create something still better. Making improvements is not limited to our physical body. They include money, friends, living in nice surroundings, going on vacation, and doing things that please us. To experience joy is what we want most, and it is easier to have joy being healthy and wealthy than being poor and sick. We want to do the things we like to do without feeling restricted. However, temporary lack may have a good side too. It awakens a desire in us to achieve something better and propels us in the right direction.

I grew up in Germany after the war, where not much of anything was available. Work and food were scarce. Luxuries were inaccessible for ordinary people. Houses in Berlin were bombed and people suffered, trying to get by. As a child, I was not aware of the tremendous lack people suffered, and in a way, I was fortunate. My grandfather had a huge garden which provided food for the whole family. He had fruit trees, vegetables, potatoes, berries, nuts, asparagus, and corn. My grandmother took care of the flowers in the front yard, and right next to the entrance to the garden were two huge jasmine bushes, which I remember well for their fragrance. A little brook was running through the back part of the garden, and an old army tank with rain water next to a compost pile served as a pool for us children. Otherwise, we had no toys. The only meat we got was once in awhile when one of the chickens was killed. We had five of them and I knew each one of them by name. I used to feed them with grass and corn, and it took me a while to understand that there was a relationship between the chicken soup we ate and one of the chickens disappearing.

My clothes were handed down to me from a distant cousin. Sometimes her mother even sent me underwear, probably thinking how happy I would be to wear it. It was nothing but humiliating. A kindhearted farmer's wife had the idea to knit some coarse, itchy knickers from sheep's wool for me to keep me warm. Not only were they itchy, they went down to my knees and looked awful. It is hard to imagine the shame I felt when one of the girls at school lifted my skirt and they were in plain sight to everybody.

It is a chapter of my life that belongs to the past. Then there was disease. As a child, I had a bout of polio, which fortunately was discovered in time and completely healed. Both my parents were heavy smokers and very sick. They suffered from the ravages of the war. My father came back home after having been prisoner in a war camp. His life was never the same again. He survived breast cancer and struggled to survive. My mother was raped and afterwards became partially paralyzed. She completely depended on my father. All this awakened a desire in me to not have a life similar to theirs. At school, I had good grades and if it had not been for the fruit and vegetables from my grandfather's garden in my earlier years, I might have been much sicker.

After I finished school, I was on my own and struggled financially because my parents could hardly support themselves, much less send me money for studies abroad. I lived on the cheapest possible food and candy bars. Whether those experiences had something to do with it or not, I do not know. In 1965, I collapsed on a street in Mexico City due to unidentified causes. Thereafter I started my search for health and a better life.

The learning never ends, and everything happens for a reason. Our greatest difficulties can turn into our greatest blessings. Each difficulty, each challenge, is given to us not as a punishment, but rather as an opportunity to learn from the situation and grow. The first step may be to recognize that we have a problem, and if it is beyond our capabilities to take care of it, ask for help. God or the Universe or whatever you call it, will respond. Some people believe in Angels. I used to think that God only speaks to a few selected persons and in a loud audible voice, especially when the preacher at church repeatedly proclaimed that "last night God spoke to him." God speaks to all of us, maybe not in a loud voice coming from Heaven but rather through thoughts, events, situations, people, ideas and opportunities. He always answers and we need to be willing to follow the leads. It is good to have knowledge and plans, and maybe even faith. However, without action nothing is going to change.

No desire is unimportant. Let's say you want more money to buy a new car. Perhaps the Universe responds by offering you a job or somebody wants to sell you a car at a price you can afford. The car is not going to appear on its own. At least you have to go to a dealer or look for advertisements in the papers. If you pray for better health, try eating less and more natural food. I am not saying that the natural way is the only way to go. In some instances, we need medical attention. Whatever the answer may be, take appropriate action. If you are not sure what to do, wait until you have more information and in case of doubt, don't do! You might want to get a second opinion first or find out whether there are other options. If you act too hasty, you might have regrets later and some interventions are irreversible.

Whether it is health or money we want or a better relationship, there is always a way to get our heart's desires. Sometimes it might be necessary to change first before our desires can manifest. If you have doubts, wait for guidance. Trust God, He always has a solution. The next step is usually right in front of you.

Besides good health, most of us would like to have a nice home, a reliable car, and money in the bank. We would like to travel, go on vacation and enjoy a few luxuries in life. Nothing is impossible. Perhaps we need to take classes on investment strategies or get more job training or education first. At the Unity Church we say, If it is to be, it is up to me! It means that God works through us. We have to take action and not just wait for our wishes to be fulfilled without our participation.

Something important to remember is that there is nothing free in the Universe. What does it mean? It means we have to give. In order to receive, we have to give. It is the law. We can give money, loving, our time, or share our talents. Whatever we give will come back to us multiplied. One of the most important blessings I received was a note from a classmate at school. She wrote in my album: "All the joy you give will come back into our own heart." So true!

Whom do we give to? If you give money, it is suggested to give at least 10 percent of our income. Churches recommend supporting them with your tithe or at least give it to the source where you receive your spiritual food. There is nothing wrong with it. I believe we can give to anybody, because we are giving back to God. Money can do a lot of good. It is energy. The key to having more is in giving more. Share with people who are less fortunate. Give to your church or to your favorite charity. Give to friends, people you know and people you don't know. Give to the poor and give to the rich. You can give money, flowers, time, food, books, or service. It does not matter. Give! It is all energy. It is a form of love. Everything you give, you give to God. Give of what you want more of.

If you want more joy, bring joy into the life of others. If you want love, be more loving. Everybody needs more love and joy in their lives. There is no need to be poor first. Whatever you give from your heart will be returned to you multiplied. Don't expect it to come back to you from the same person you gave to but when you give without expecting anything in return, you will be rewarded. It is the fastest way to be blessed and grow rich. As a result of giving you may be blessed with better health or peace of mind. There is no need to work harder or chase the good things. Prosperity will find you.

Whatever we give, we are always giving to God, even if we give to ourselves. We are all God's children. The wealthier we are, the more we have to share. When you tithe to yourself, you can buy goods or services with the money, or you can offer a job to somebody and pay them generously. Most people would rather have an opportunity to earn money than depend on handouts or charity. This way, you are both blessed: Somebody has an opportunity to have an income and you choose what you want in return.

There is a beautiful story about an Indian Saint by the name of Guru Nanak: One day Guru Nanak was in a temple with his feet pointing towards the altar. One of the worshippers reprimanded him, telling him that it was a sacrilege to point his feet in the direction of God. The Saint replied, "Show me any place where God is not, and that is where I will put my feet."

Whether rich or poor, everybody would like more love in their lives. We can give our love by sharing our blessings. We may give of our time, money, or talents. Fasting is a way of giving as well. It is probably the fastest way to achieve better health. Since we are going to get something in return, we may just as well tell the Universe what it is we would like or pray for it. We are never alone. There are always angels around us who hear our prayers even if we don't see them with our physical eyes. Maybe God Himself is waiting for a request and ready to give us whatever we ask for, or something better. His answer may come in the form of a thought, a book, a person, or something happening. Everything is a learning experience and whatever we give out, good or bad, will come back to us. It is called the law of karma. Challenges are opportunities to grow.

When people change their diets and see results, even after nothing else has worked for them before, they feel blessed. I surely appreciate good thoughts but God is the one in charge. Healers can only provide us with guidance. We still have to do our part. Our body is such an incredible and perfect mechanism that it heals itself when we know how to give it the proper care. When I was sick and no medical doctor could do anything for me, Dr. Sperl healed me with herbs and diet. He did not take credit for it. In his infinite wisdom, he only said: "IT IS MOTHER NATURE WHO DOES THE HEALING. WE ONLY HAVE TO GIVE HER A HAND." God provides us with everything we need, but we have to do our part to receive the blessings.

All choices we make have consequences. They can be as simple as choosing between eating and not eating, between walking or staying at home and watching TV, between being aware of the needs of others or thinking of ourselves. We receive in the proportion of our giving, and invisible friends are always anxious to help us. They can be angels or loved ones in Spirit. It could be a Master, a teacher or a healer on the other side. We do not know. Just act as if there was no doubt in your mind about their existence and ask for help. These loving and powerful beings are there for you. Thank them in advance for what you want and it will be done, always adding: "This or something better, if it is for my highest good."

If you think you have nothing to give, you can still count your blessings. Be grateful for what you already have. Actually, it is the fastest way to experience wealth and attract more good in your life. Be grateful for the roof over your head, for friends, sunshine, the rain, your job, a pet, your car starting in the morning, food, the beauty of nature, good health, a kindness somebody extended to you, or your next breath. Life itself is the greatest gift. We all have something to be grateful for because there are many who are less fortunate.

Instead of being concerned about what we don't have, we can either be grateful for what we do have or share with those who have less. Actually, the one that gives is the one that receives the most. To be able to give is the greatest blessing. The secret to a healthy, prosperous life is to love more and give more, because the blessings already are. They only become visible along the way.

Have a happy journey!

Acknowledgements

I express my gratitude to everybody who contributed to the making of this book, too many to mention by name. I thank those who inspired me, sometimes with a cry for help or the learning that came from it. I thank my most wonderful, outstanding teachers: Dr. Juan Sperl, Swami Pranavananda Saraswati, and John-Roger, as well as my spiritual guides.

I thank my editor Alethea Spiridon, Pia Jameson at Balboa Press and everybody who helped in some way in getting this book published. Carlos, my love, inspired me to ever new discoveries and gave me opportunities to grow. I am also grateful to Rev. Diana Isaac and Rev. Leiris Morillo from Unity El Paso, who were always there for me with unconditional love and support.

I very much appreciate the endorsement by Dr. Terry Cole-Whittaker, famous best-selling author, teacher, minister, spiritual counselor and therapist: "The contents of KISS YOUR DOCTOR GOODBYE has been well researched and is presented in an easy to understand way. If you want a healthy, vibrant body and life, then read this book! An intelligent person always retains responsibility for his or her own life, especially their health. Besides having a good health advisor one needs to know what is possible. This book is a great resource for yourself and your family."

Finally, I thank you, the reader, for being part of my life, for your willingness to look into dietary changes and natural therapies and apply them when appropriate. May you be blessed above all, with good health. Between all of us we create a better world. My spiritual teacher, John-Roger, would say: **The blessings already are.** We are the blessings, each one of us.

Recommended Reading and Videos

by some of the greatest teachers:

Armstrong, J.W.: The Water of Life
by C.W. Daniel Co. Ltd., England, 1971

Boutenko, Victoria: Green for Life
by Raw Family Publishing, Canada, 2005

Bragg, Paul: Healthy Lifestyle & The Miracle of Fasting
by Bragg Health Crusades/Health Science, California

Brandt, Johanna: The Grape Cure
by Ehret Literature Publishing Co., New York, around 1927

Christy, Martha: Your Own Perfect Medicine
by Self Healing Press, Arizona, 1994

Dr. Crook, William: The Yeast Connection
by Square One, USA, 2007

Cross, Joe: Fat, Sick and Nearly Dead
documentary 2010

Diamond, Harvey &   Fit For Life
Marilyn:
by Warner Books, Inc., New York, 1985

Dufty, William: The Sugar Blues
by Warner Books, Pennsylvania, 1975

Ehret, Arnold: The Musucsless Diet Healing System
by Ehret Literature Company, New York, 1953, 1981, 1983,
1994

Escher, Ursula: A Day in the Budwig Diet
by UEscher Productions, USA,2011

Jensen, Bernard: The Chemistry of Man
by Bernard Jensen, California, 1983

John-Roger: Wealth and Higher Consciousness
by Mandeville Press, Los Angeles, CA., 1988

Mosley, Michael: Eat, Fast and Live Longer
documentary 2014

Muhammad, Elijah: How to Eat to Live (book 2)
by Secretaris MEMPS Publications, Arizona, 1972

National   Blue Zones, The Science of Living
Geographic: Longer
by National Geographic Partners, Washington, 2016

Openshaw, Robyn: Vibe
by North Star Way, New York, 2017

Oshawa, George (Sakurazawa Nyoiti): You are all Sampaku, by University Books, USA, 1965

Osho: From Medication to Meditation by C.W. Daniel Co. Ltd., SA, 1994

Rothkranz, Markus: Vegan Strongman Eats Only One Meal a Day documentary, 2016 interview with Dr. Nun Amen-Ra

Dr. Shinya, Hiromi: The Microbe Factor by Millichap Books, San Francisco, 2010

Dr. Simoncini, Tullius: Cancer is a Fungus by Edizioni Lampos, Italy, 2007

Sinclair, Upton: The Fasting Cure by William Heinemann, London, 1911

Spurlock, Morgan: Supersize Me documentary 2004

Wilde, Stuart: The Force by Hayhouse, California, 1997

Wolfe, David: Eating for Beauty by North Atlantic Books, Berkely, CA. 2007, 2009

Zavasta, Tonya: Quantum Eating, the Ultimate Elixir of Youth by BR Publishing LLC, Tennessee, 2012

In Spanish:

Capo, Nicolas: Mis Observaciones Clinicas sobre el Limon, el Ajo y la Cebolla
by Editorial Kier, Buenos Aires, 1966

Lezaeta A., Manuel: La Medicina Natural al Alcance de Todos
Editorial Pax, Mexico, 1956

Mazdaznan: EnciclopediaNaturista, Serie No. 7
by Mazdaznan Press Los Angles, Ca. 1970
traducido al español, e imprimido en Mexico, 1974

Dr. Pros, Miguel: Como Cura la Avena (Healing with Oats)
by Dr. Miguel Pros y RBA Libros, S.A., Barcelona, 2012

In French:

Simoneton, André: Radiations des Aliments, Ondes Humaine et Santé
by Le Courrier du Libre, Paris, 1971

In German:

Nissim, Rina;   Naturheilkunde in der Gynaekologie
by Orlanda Frauenverlag, Germany, 1984

References: * The Bible - New King James' Version,
© 1979, 1980, 1982,
by permission of Thomas Nelson, Inc., USA

About the Author

Elke Lewis is a Traditional Naturopath and Nutritionist with over 40 years in private practice. Over the years, she has helped thousands of people to recuperate their health, mainly through nutrition. Ms. Lewis studied yoga and some of the secrets of Eastern healing techniques with a Master from India, and has degrees in Nutrition from Germany, the U.S., and South America. She is also an ordained minister in M.S.I.A.

In her book KISS YOUR DOCTOR GOODBYE she reveals all natural methods to achieve lasting health without the need for complicated or costly procedures. She includes the stories of people who made a few simple changes in their lifestyle and got a new lease on life. Some wanted to lose extra pounds, others to improve their eyesight, to become pregnant after failed efforts, to normalize their blood sugar or blood pressure, or to recover from "incurable" diseases. Others decided to turn the clock back and look and feel young again. She believes that natural cures never disappoint anyone. As long as you do your part, the way you feel and look afterwards might pleasantly surprise you.

Printed in the United States
By Bookmasters